Neurology - Laboratory and Clinical
Research Developments

Manual of Spinal Endoscopy

A New Method for the Diagnosis and Therapy of Chronic Spinal Pain

NEUROLOGY - LABORATORY AND CLINICAL RESEARCH DEVELOPMENTS

Additional books in this series can be found on Nova's website under the Series tab.

Additional e-books in this series can be found on Nova's website under the e-book tab.

NEUROLOGY - LABORATORY AND CLINICAL
RESEARCH DEVELOPMENTS

MANUAL OF SPINAL ENDOSCOPY

A NEW METHOD FOR THE DIAGNOSIS AND THERAPY OF CHRONIC SPINAL PAIN

DIEGO BELTRUTTI
EDITOR

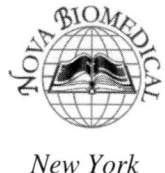

New York

Copyright © 2012 by Nova Science Publishers, Inc.

All rights reserved. No part of this book may be reproduced, stored in a retrieval system or transmitted in any form or by any means: electronic, electrostatic, magnetic, tape, mechanical photocopying, recording or otherwise without the written permission of the Publisher.

For permission to use material from this book please contact us:
Telephone 631-231-7269; Fax 631-231-8175
Web Site: http://www.novapublishers.com

NOTICE TO THE READER

The Publisher has taken reasonable care in the preparation of this book, but makes no expressed or implied warranty of any kind and assumes no responsibility for any errors or omissions. No liability is assumed for incidental or consequential damages in connection with or arising out of information contained in this book. The Publisher shall not be liable for any special, consequential, or exemplary damages resulting, in whole or in part, from the readers' use of, or reliance upon, this material. Any parts of this book based on government reports are so indicated and copyright is claimed for those parts to the extent applicable to compilations of such works.

Independent verification should be sought for any data, advice or recommendations contained in this book. In addition, no responsibility is assumed by the publisher for any injury and/or damage to persons or property arising from any methods, products, instructions, ideas or otherwise contained in this publication.

This publication is designed to provide accurate and authoritative information with regard to the subject matter covered herein. It is sold with the clear understanding that the Publisher is not engaged in rendering legal or any other professional services. If legal or any other expert assistance is required, the services of a competent person should be sought. FROM A DECLARATION OF PARTICIPANTS JOINTLY ADOPTED BY A COMMITTEE OF THE AMERICAN BAR ASSOCIATION AND A COMMITTEE OF PUBLISHERS.

Additional color graphics may be available in the e-book version of this book.

Library of Congress Cataloging-in-Publication Data

ISBN: 978-1-62257-250-2
Library of Congress Control Number: 2012940316

Published by Nova Science Publishers, Inc. † New York

Contents

Foreword		vii
Introduction		ix
Abbreviations		xi
Chapter 1	Features of Spinal Endoscopy *Fabio Intelligente*	1
Chapter 2	The Spinal Endoscope *Diego Beltrutti*	5
Chapter 3	Techniques of Endoscopy *Diego Beltrutti*	9
Chapter 4	Anatomical Significance of the Spinal Canal *Diego Beltrutti*	13
Chapter 5	Epiduroscopic Diagnosis *Diego Beltrutti*	17
Chapter 6	The Fibrosis of the Epidural Space *Lorenzo Pasquariello*	19
Chapter 7	Patient Evaluation *Diego Beltrutti*	25
Chapter 8	Indications *Diego Beltrutti*	31
Chapter 9	Key Aspects of the Technique *Diego Beltrutti*	37

Chapter 10	Recognizing Endoscopic Images *Attilio Di Donato*	45
Chapter 11	After the Procedure *Diego Beltrutti*	53
Chapter 12	Maintaining Sterility *Diego Beltrutti*	57
Chapter 13	Contraindications *Attilio Di Donato*	63
Chapter 14	Complications *Diego Beltrutti*	67
Chapter 15	Perioperative Management of Thromboprophylaxis and Antithrombotic Therapy *Fabio Intelligente*	77
Chapter 16	The Risk of Spinal Hematoma *Lorenzo Pasquariello*	83
Chapter 17	Historical Considerations *Diego Beltrutti*	87
Chapter 18	Consensus Conference on Spinal Endoscopy *Diego Beltrutti*	101
Chapter 19	Essential Equipment *Diego Beltrutti*	107
Chapter 20	Materials *Attilio Di Donato*	113
Chapter 21	Future Trends *Diego Beltrutti*	119
Chapter 22	Conclusion *Diego Beltrutti*	123
References		125
Acknowledgments		135
Contributors		137
Index		139

Foreword

Among the most interesting and difficult challenges that a doctor can undertake is surely the treatment of patients with persistent and chronic pain syndromes. These conditions not only result in physical exhaustion and have a psychological impact on the patient, but are also important from the social and societal perspectives. In this field of medicine a very important focus is on chronic pain of the spine, with a disease component that is commonly referred to as "biopsychosocial".

While a variety of therapeutic options exist for the treatment of chronic spinal pain, the availability of these options is often dependent on culture or beliefs, as well as the training and skills of the treating clinician. Currently, the diagnosis of persistent pain conditions of the spine is by no means standardized, and there has been a lack of clear consensus regarding appropriate algorithms both for diagnosis and for treatment. One needs only to recall the case of discography, which was recognized as having diagnostic value but of uncertain applicability in routine clinical practice.

There are several reasons for these uncertainties including an absence of guidelines that are mutually accepted by different communities of specialists, and only a limited number of schools specializing in pain medicine. The lack of recognition at the university level of pain medicine as a medical specialty area is another factor that plays a negative role.

All these reasons contribute to a narrow perspective, lacking the focus and objectives required for advancing diagnostic and treatment paradigms. In fact, in order to determine the correct indication for a patient with chronic spinal pain, it is required to define the cause of the pain through a process that is not structured and has not been standardized.

An important component of diagnosis and treatment of chronic spinal pain, at least for the most complex and difficult cases, is the procedure of spinal endoscopy, a minimally invasive endoscopic technique recently introduced for use in clinical practice. It allows the direct identification of pathological states present in the epidural space, and can also be used for targeted pharmacotherapy to ameliorate the pathological processes that trigger the pain.

Although studies on spinal endoscopy present in the international medical literature are still limited and evidences are often linked to the personal experience of pain physicians it seems that there is a growing interest of the scientific community towards this technique. Recent publications are validating the utility of this procedure and broadening acceptance of its effectiveness for both diagnosis and therapy. It can be expected that the specific roles of this procedure will be defined relative to other invasive and non-invasive therapeutic procedures, and its cost-benefit ratio will be assessed to better characterize areas of application.

The challenge for its clinical acceptance is to provide the medical evidence showing that consistent results are obtained when clinicians performing this procedure have appropriate educational training and accreditation, and use standardized quality instrumentation as part of defined protocols.

Introduction

Why this manual on "Spinal Endoscopy"? Because we felt that it is currently necessary for those who have dedicated themselves to the study and practice of Pain Medicine to make their voices heard to an audience that encompasses a broad range of physicians who may benefit from such knowledge.

In recent years, technological advances have resulted in the development of sophisticated and innovative tools and equipment for "minimally invasive" pain management. Gaining the knowledge and ability to effectively use these tools involves a learning curve that is neither easy nor quick.

Thus, there is a problem of where to learn these new procedures. Individual companies responsible for developing these technologies have made a considerable effort in training specialist physicians by sending them to workshops that have provided a theoretical foundation as well as practical experience using cadavers. Nevertheless, practical experience is still limited, and may also be flawed by poor understanding by the participants if the workshop is in a non-native language of the participants.

Over the last ten years there has been a growing interest in pain. The neurophysiological knowledge has grown and promising new drugs have been introduced to treat chronic pain states. The medical literature has seen the publication of encyclopaedic texts published by scientific societies, famous universities and internationally renowned specialists; bulky volumes that are useful for those approaching the subject as they deal with all aspects from indications to complications and including anatomy, psychology, physiology and pharmacology.

Some specialist monographs that systematically and comprehensively address the primary minimally invasive analgesic techniques have been published here and there but these are works that are often difficult to find.

Globally, there are situations in which the training of new interventional pain techniques are entrusted to device manufacturers. This can be accepted up to a certain extent.

The theoretical teaching and practical experience made on cadavers together with the evaluation of knowledge and skills acquired in percutaneous pain procedures is therefore a crucial fact. Scientific societies have played a lot of work together with universities in the dissemination of an increasingly safer practice of pain medicine.

In our country, Italy, we therefore thought to support the online training courses that the Italian School of Pain Medicine (SIMED) has prepared in the past nine years with a series of texts to guide physicians-in-training and to act as a review for established clinicians for providing a stepwise approach to a deeper understanding of the theory and practice of specific techniques. The realization of this handbook on spinal endoscopy is born from that experience and collaboration with SIMED and the Italian College of Pain Physicians (CIMA).

In the realization and editing of this first book, I relied on the help of Dr. Attilio Di Donato, Dr. Fabio Intelligente and Dr. Lorenzo Pasquariello, pain physicians with long and recognized experience in spinal endoscopy.

Diego Beltrutti, MD, FIPP, CIMA

Director, Italian School of Pain Medicine (SIMED)
Past President World Society of Pain Clinicians (WSPS)
Pain Service, Istituti Clinici Humanitas, Rozzano (Mi), Italy

Abbreviations

Some of the following abbreviations are used in this text and/or commonly encountered in the literature in the case of endoscopic procedures and spinal pain.

CHF	Congestive Heart Failure
CNB	Central Neuraxial Block
CNS	Central Nervous System
COPD	Chronic Obstructive Pulmonary Disease
CSF	Cerebro Spinal Fluid
CT	Computerized Tomography
DCS	Day Case Surgery
PDD	Percutaneous Disc Decompression, a mechanical intradiscal procedure based on insertion of a motorized needle into the nucleus pulposus and subsequent removal of material from the nucleus pulposus
DRG	Dorsal Root Ganglia
DVT	Deep Vein Thrombosis
EKG or ECG	Electro Cardiography
EGD	Esophageal Gastric Duodenoscopy; direct visualization of the mucosa of the esophagus, stomach and duodenum using a flexible fiberoptic scope
EMG	Electro Myography
ERCP	Endoscopic Retrograde Cholangio Pancreatography

ESC	Endoscopy of the Spinal Canal
FBSS	Failed Back Surgery Syndrome. FBSS is a nonspecific term referring to a lack of benefit following one or more low back surgeries
IDD	Internal Disc Disruption
IDET	Intra Discal Electro Thermal annuloplasty
INR	International Normalized Ratio
LBP	Low Back Pain
LMWH	Low Molecular Weight Heparin
MRI	Magnetic Resonance Imaging
MRCP	Magnetic Resonance Cholangio Pancreatography
NCV	Nerve Conduction Velocity
NIBP	Not Invasive Blood Pressure
NSAIDs	Non Steroidal Anti Inflammatory Drugs
ODS	One-Day Surgery; the patient is staying in the hospital at least overnight
PDPH	Post Dural Puncture Headache
PE	Pulmonary Embolism
PLDD	Percutaneous Laser Disc Decompression
PR or BPM	Pulse Rate or Beats Per Minute
QST	Quantitative Sensory Testing; neurophysiologic examination that evaluates specifically nerve fibers of the C, A-delta, and A-beta types
RF	Radiofrequency. A group of minimally invasive pain procedures using the thermal and electrical effect of radio frequencies
SCS	Spinal Cord Stimulation
SE	Spinal Endoscopy
SEH	Spinal Epidural Hematoma
Single shot	Literally: "a single injection". It can refer to a spinal or epidural injection in contrast to the continuous administration through a spinal or epidural catheter
SpO2	Saturation of Peripheral Oxygen
SSEP	Somato Sensory Evoked Potentials
TDBA	Trans Discal Bi-Accuplasty

VTD	Venous Thromboembolic Disease
VGC	Video Guided Catheter
WSCM	Water Soluble Contrast Media; ionic monomers, ionic dimmers or non ionic monomers can be used. Metrizamide and Iopamidol belong to this last group.

In: Manual of Spinal Endoscopy
Editor: Diego Beltrutti

ISBN: 978-1-62257-250-2
© 2012 Nova Science Publishers, Inc.

Chapter 1

Features of Spinal Endoscopy

Fabio Intelligente
Chronic Pain Service, Istituti Clinici Humanitas,
Rozzano (MI), Italy
Italian School of Pain Medicine (SIMED), Italy

Spinal Endoscopy (SE), also known as Periduroscopy or Epiduroscopy, is a procedure that consists of the percutaneous placement of a flexible fiber optic endoscope into the epidural space through the sacral hiatus. This technique enables direct visualization of anatomical structures present in the epidural space including the dura mater, nerves, blood vessels, connective tissue, and adipose tissue.

Spinal endoscopy also allows the injection of pharmacologic agents in a targeted manner, thus mechanically helping the expansion and the opening up of the epidural space. This action can possibly disperse adhesions and fibroses that may be present and contribute to, or are the cause of persistent spinal pain.

Spinal endoscopy is a percutaneous, minimally invasive technique that has recently become more widely available for a variety of applications. It has proven to be a valuable diagnostic aid because it allows direct visualization of pathologic abnormalities in the epidural space such as inflammation, adhesions, scars, fibrosis and stenotic changes within the spinal canal.

SE is also a valid therapeutic procedure for removing the adhesions and scar tissue that may be responsible for maintaining a state of nerve root irritation. Subsequent to other techniques that include epidural blocks using single shot or continuous infusion through a dedicated epidural catheter (for example: Gold-Kath®, Tun-L-Cath® or similar), electrical neurostimulation (Spinal Cord Stimulation or SCS from Medtronic, St Jude, Boston Scientific), implanted pumps for continuous intrathecal administration (Codman, Medtronic, Bard), radiofrequency procedures of the anulus (IDET, TDBA) or nucleus pulposus (Nucleoplasty, Reliefer, Dekompressor, PLDD), pain clinicians are finally learning to exploit the advantages of endoscopic techniques.

It can be observed that SE has become an exciting and noteworthy technique for diagnosis and therapy that continues to become of greater clinical relevance for patients with persistent and chronic pain originating from the lumbar sacral segment. This growth in interest of SE has come about due to greater education of clinicians and the development of more technologically advanced equipment that uses flexible endoscopes that have been increasingly miniaturized while increasing optical resolution.

Since SE is a minimally invasive procedure, it has several advantages:

- pain is limited, both during and after the procedure
- short monitoring time after procedure
- the duration of convalescence is short
- in the absence of complications a delayed return to work can not be attributed to the procedure since there is no surgical involvement of bones, ligaments or muscles.

With endoscopy, medical science has succeeded in realizing the very old dream of observing the human body from within. To date, there have only been limited methods that allowed visual survey of the interior of a patient or an organ, some using surgical procedures, and others enabling evaluation of specific body cavities using specialized equipment.

Optical fiber technology has become sufficiently advanced that through the use of very thin fibers it can now be applied to "minimally invasive" percutaneous procedures capable of transmitting an image of good definition. These advances enable direct visualization of the inner surface of body cavities and organs including the spinal canal.

This procedure, which is called "endoscopy" (literally "see inside") is based on using an instrument called an endoscope and has most commonly been applied for techniques of:

- Gastroscopy: an investigational procedure for visualization and/or histological sampling (biopsy) of the stomach.
- Proctoscopy and colonoscopy: an examination that enables viewing of the last part of the large intestine.
- Laparoscopy: a technique to examine the abdominal cavity and perform surgical interventions such as appendectomies, cholecystectomies, colectomies, etc.
- Arthroscopy: a procedure for exploring the interior of a joint and performing endoscopic surgical interventions.

More recently, spinal endoscopy has entered the field as a minimally invasive technique in which the endoscopic instrument is inserted percutaneously through an incision of 0.5 cm, performed under local anesthesia at the sacral hiatus. This allows not only exploration and evaluation of the lower lumbar and sacral epidural space, but also an ability to perform therapeutic procedures such as lysis of epidural adhesions according to the method of Racz, carrying out of epidural biopsies and precise placement of electrodes for SCS.

Endoscopy can be accomplished by either a rigid or flexible endoscope. In this manual we will only report about spinal endoscopy performed with a flexible endoscope.

The epiduroscope used for caudal endoscopy is of the flexible type, consisting of a tube carrying very thin optical fibers capable of channeling light energy generated by an external source to the tip of the endoscope. Other fibers are appointed to convey the image that comes from the epidural space to the external monitor.

Spinal endoscopy is a medical procedure that has become of considerable importance, especially in cases where there are discrepancies between the information obtained from standard imaging techniques such as X-rays, CT and MRI, clinical evaluation and neuro physiological tests such as EMG and SSEP. In contrast to these techniques, endoscopy not only provides images of the anatomical structures in the segment we want to examine, but also allows us to perform biopsies, lysis of epidural adhesions, and the targeted placement of dedicated epidural catheters or electrodes for SCS in specific anatomical areas difficult to reach.

Clinical research and experimental models have already given, and will continue to give new impetus to this technology and the resulting procedures for diagnosis and endoscopic surgery. Furthermore, the possibility of endoscopically inserting probes and micro-instruments such as lasers or RF will additionally drive the development and acceptance of these techniques and expand their possibilities for clinical use.

This technology is able to offer increasingly flexible endoscopes of smaller diameter and greater versatility, which enable images of increased quality. These advances can be expected to improve safety and result in a greater acceptance among clinicians and patients.

Clearly the information that a pain clinician can collect through a direct vision of the epidural nerve structures, is greater than that which can be obtained through a mental reconstruction of MRI, CT, EMG data and clinical evaluation.

Improvements in percutaneous microsurgical techniques have enabled specialists to become more efficient and better able to document complex pathological states because of their new-found ability to visually record the procedures carried out. This is also an invaluable contribution to forensic medicine.

1.1. Terminology Issues

The original term used to define endoscopic evaluation of the epidural space, attributed to Rune Blomberg, was "epiduroscopy." In the U.S. there was a reluctance by insurance companies to reimburse epiduroscopy procedures, since they had no familiarity with the term and it did not appear in the books of coding procedures provided to insurance companies.

While insurance officials did not know where to place epiduroscopy, everything became easier when it was called spinal endoscopy. This new procedure fell well within the framework of endoscopy, and the term "endoscopy of the spinal canal" or ESC was adopted because of familiarity with endoscopy in the U.S. insurance market.

Today the term endoscopy of the spinal canal or simply spinal endoscopy refers to both Epiduroscopy, evaluation by a flexible fiber optic instrument (endoscope) positioned in the epidural space, and to Myeloscopy, which is a method of direct visualization of the subarachnoid structures.

In: Manual of Spinal Endoscopy
Editor: Diego Beltrutti

ISBN: 978-1-62257-250-2
© 2012 Nova Science Publishers, Inc.

Chapter 2

The Spinal Endoscope

Diego Beltrutti
Chronic Pain Service, Istituti Clinici Humanitas,
Rozzano (MI), Italy
Italian School of Pain Medicine (SIMED), Italy

Spinal Endoscopy is a procedure used to diagnose the causes of chronic radicular back pain. It is a minimally invasive pain procedure that is based on the insertion of an instrument called "spinal endoscope" that, using a flexible fiberoptic endoscope and a steerable video guided catheter allows the inspection of the epidural space[1].

Spinal endoscopes have different outside diameters that are generally not greater than 3.5 mm, and have a working channel ranging from 0.9 mm to 1.5 mm. Through a system of proximal magnification, images are obtained using a lens system, resulting in excellent image quality even at focal distances smaller than one millimeter. The lens is connected to a camera system that can make a permanent record of what is visualized during the procedure.

The instruments use a digitized system in which the image is transferred via microprocessors to obtain a color image. This takes place directly through the camera head, allowing for optimal contrast and resolution.

---

[1] In this session are listed personal judgments on some of the individual flexible spinal endoscopes available on the market. These judgments reflect the personal and sincere opinions of the authors. These opinions do not want to be an invitation to use one tool over another. There are no secondary factors in defining of these judgments.

A variety of flexible epiduroscopes are currently available internationally, having different technical characteristics that, although similar, are not identical. Are now described the features and short reviews on the spinal endoscopy systems more easily available on the market. Judgements expressed here by the authors are personal, genuine and are not resulting from economic ties, consulting contracts or whatever.

Myelotec Video Guided Catheter. (VGC). This instrument has been developed by Myelotec (Myelotec, Atlanta, Georgia). It is a disposable video guide consisting of a non-traumatic radiopaque plastic material with a good bi-directional guide. The Myelotec VGC is used in combination with a reusable flexible optical fiber endoscope that has to be re-sterilized in order to be reused. This VGC is available in two sizes, 2.7 mm (8 Fr) and 3.0 mm (9 Fr) outer diameters. Among other features has a soft, atraumatic tip, radiopaque shaft, dual infusion ports and two operating channels. The kit contains all the mechanical components that enable caudal access.

Clarus Spine Scope. This instrument has been developed by Clarus (Clarus Medical System, Minneapolis, Minnesota). Compared to the Myelotec VGC, the Clarus Spine Scope has a harder body with a relatively blunt distal tip. The outside diameter is 2,3 mm. The steerable endoscope tip allows only one a single direction of deflection (up to 45°). The Spine Scope has excellent optics, a viewing angle of 70°, and a working channel that allows the use of tools up to 1 mm in diameter. It is also totally "disposable" for ease of use.

Myelotec NaviCath. This is a steerable epidural catheter having a diameter of 1.7 mm (5 Fr) thus allowing it to be introduced using a simple Tuohy needle with a 15 gauge introducer. This is used only for targeted administration of medications within the lower spinal column.

Karl Storz Epiduroscope (KSE). This instrument has been developed by Karl Storz (Karl Storz, Tuttlingen, Germany). It is a classic endoscope indicated for use in the lumbar and sacral spine for observing epidural anathomy and pathology. It is available in different lengths (40 and 70 cm). The cord is flexible, has an outer diameter of 2.8 mm, and incorporates a working channel with a diameter of 1.2 mm. The distal tip can be directed up or down at an angle between 120° and 170°.

Karl Storz Miniature Epiduroscope. This instrument has an outside diameter of 0.5 mm. It has been designed only for diagnostic purposes. It can be used as epiduroscope but also as spinaloscope. The main feature of this endoscope is the very high flexibility. It presents an angle vision of 0° and an opening angle of 55°.

Karl Storz Epiduroscope FLEX - X2. This epiduroscope is an attempt to balance the need of an improved image resolution with the size of the instrument. This epiduroscope has an outer diameter of 3,1 mm, a length of 90 cm, a visual angle of 0° and an angle of deflection of 270°. The presence of a Laserite ceramic at the distal tip guarantees protection in case of a combined laser use.

Wolf Epiduroscope. This instrument has been developed by Richard Wolf (Richard Wolf GmbH, Knittlingen, Germany). It is a flexible epidurosope that is 70 cm long. It is produced in two versions: with an outer diameter of 2.5 mm (7.5 Fr) or 3,0 cm (9 Fr). In the first one the working channel has a diameter of 1.2 mm and in the second one 1.5 mm. The distal tip can be directed up to 130° or down at an angle of 160°.

EPI-C Spinal Endoscope. This instrument has been developed by Equip Medikey (Equip Medikey, Gouda, The Netherlands). This is considered to be a good and versatile spinal endoscope. This flexible tool has an outside diameter of 2.65 mm (8 Fr), a steerable tip of 180°, a first working channel of 1.2 mm (3,6 Fr), and a second working channel 0.6 mm (1.9 Fr) that is used for irrigation. It is available in 30 cm and 60 cm lengths. The advantage of this endoscope is that the fiber optic can not get out from the tip of the endoscope by a lens that has the effect of completely isolating it from contact with the epidural space. Thus, it is not necessary to sterilize the optical fiber between procedures, limiting the need for fiber replacement since it is known that repeated sterilization damages the fibers. Among the advantages claimed by the manufacturer there is a handling fee of 30% less compared to competitors.

In: Manual of Spinal Endoscopy
Editor: Diego Beltrutti

ISBN: 978-1-62257-250-2
© 2012 Nova Science Publishers, Inc.

Chapter 3

Techniques of Endoscopy

Diego Beltrutti
Chronic Pain Service, Istituti Clinici Humanitas,
Rozzano (MI), Italy
Italian School of Pain Medicine (SIMED), Italy

Fiber optic endoscopy has now permeated the medical field and is utilized in a myriad of diagnostic and therapeutic procedures including:

Arthroscopy: viewing of the articular cavity (knee, hip, shoulder, wrist, other joints) for diagnostic and therapeutic purposes (arthroscopic meniscectomy, rotator cuff tears, frozen shoulder (adhesive capsulitis), shoulder instability, cruciate ligament surgery, femoro-acetabular impingement, etc.). From the time of Professor Kenji Takagi who has been credited for performing the first arthroscopic examination of the knee joint of a patient in 1919, we assisted to a continuous technical progress.

Bronchoscopy: examination of the trachea and the bronchial tree for diagnostic and therapeutic purposes. Bronchoscopy can reveal the presence of abscesses, bronchitis, cancer, tuberculosis, alveolitis, infection and inflammation of the upper respiratory system. A German, Gustav Killian, performed the first bronchoscopy in 1897 with a rigid bronchoscope. Rigid bronchoscopes have been used until 1966 when the Japanese Shigeto Ikeda, invented the flexible bronchoscope.

Colonoscopy: internal examination of the colon (large intestine) and rectum, using an instrument called colonoscope. This technique, now widely accepted and practiced and at the very beginning opposed, was introduced in medical practice at the end of the '60. It has diagnostic and therapeutic purposes. Colonoscopy can reveal the presence of polyps, tumors, ulcers, inflammation, ulcerative colitis, diverticulosis, Crohn's disease. This procedure can be used also for the identification and removal of foreign bodies.

Colposcopy: direct visualization of the vagina and cervix for early diagnosis of cancer, inflammation and other pathological conditions. Colposcopy was introduced by Hans Hinselmann in 1925, in Germany. He theorized that it might be possible to detect cervical cancer at an early stage by properly illuminating and magnifying the cervix.

Cystoscopy: direct visualization of the bladder, urethra, urinary tract, uterine orifices, and prostate (in males) by inserting the endoscope through the urethra. The procedure can also be used for taking biopsies for pathologic research. The presence of blood in the urine (hematury), certain symptoms in the urinary tract or the presence of urinary infections in women are the main causes for carrying out a cystoscopy. Philipp von Bozzini (1773-1809), a young German army surgeon, invented in 1807 an instrument that was the ancestor of the modern endoscope.

ERCP (Endoscopic Retrograde Cholangio Pancreatography): examination of the biliary tree, liver, gallbladder, pancreatic duct and other anatomical structures in search of calculi and other types of obstructive disease. It relies on endoscopic guidance to place a catheter into a duct for contrast imaging, and depends on the use of fluoroscopy. When ERCP detects an abnormality, it can often be treated immediately during the same session, or a biopsy can be performed to exclude cancer or other diseases.

The ERCP may show the presence of biliary cirrhosis, bile duct cancer, pancreatic cysts and pseudocysts, pancreatic tumors, chronic pancreatitis and other clinical conditions such as gallstones. The recent development of safer and relatively non-invasive investigations such as magnetic resonance cholangiopancreatography (MRCP) and endoscopic ultrasound has meant that ERCP is now rarely performed without therapeutic intent.

EGD (Esophageal Gastric Duodenoscopy): visual examination of the upper intestinal tract. It allows excellent visualization of the esophagus, stomach (gastric area) and the first part of the duodenum (the first segment of the small intestine). This procedure is widely used for the diagnosis of bleeding, gastric ulcers, hiatal hernia, esophagitis, gastritis, pre cancerous lesions.

Endoscopic biopsy: the removal of tissue samples for pathologic analysis and evaluation, and is carried out during different endoscopic procedures.

Laparoscopy: direct visualization of the stomach, liver and other abdominal organs including female reproductive organs (e.g. the fallopian tubes). It is an operation performed in the abdomen or pelvis through small incisions (usually 0.5–1.5 cm) with the aid of a camera. It can either be used to inspect and diagnose a condition or to perform surgery. Today more and more colectomies, nefrectomies, colecistecthomies, inguinal hernia repairs, etc. are performed in video laparoscopy.

Laryngoscopy: direct visual examination of the larynx. The idea started in the nineteenth century when Benjamin Guy Babington (1794–1866), proposed his "glottiscope". Philipp von Bozzini and Garignard de la Tour were other pioneers in the direct inspection of oropharynx and hypopharynx based on the use of mirrors. Today modern technology offers us fiberoptic and video laryngoscopes. These devices incorporate a high resolution digital camera, connected by a video cable to a high resolution LCD monitor. Laringoscopes can be used for tracheal intubation as well as for removal of foreign bodies from the airway providing, at the same time, controlled mechanical ventilation.

Proctoscopy, Sigmoidoscopy, Proctosigmoidoscopy: internal visual examination of the anus and lower part of the rectum (Proctoscopy). When the exam deals with sigmoid colon the procedure is called sigmoidoscopy. During screening flexible sigmoidoscopy it is possible to detect and intervene on small polyps.

Thoracoscopy: examination of the pleural cavity, mediastinum and pericardium. It consists in the insertion of a video endoscope through a very small incision (cut) in the chest wall. This technique allows a direct vision of the lungs or other structures of the chest cavity. Thoracoscopy can be used to collect tissue samples to diagnose lung cancer or mesothelioma (thoracoscopic biopsy). It can be used to remove a portion of the lung (thoracoscopic wedge resection or thoracoscopic lobectomy).

"Wireless" Capsule Endoscopy: pill-size video capsules enable "wireless" endoscopy and represent a newly introduced diagnostic tool, useful for diagnosing small bowel diseases as the video capsule travels through the digestive tract. However, this technique is still not widely used in clinical practice.

In: Manual of Spinal Endoscopy
Editor: Diego Beltrutti
ISBN: 978-1-62257-250-2
© 2012 Nova Science Publishers, Inc.

Chapter 4

Anatomical Significance of the Spinal Canal

Diego Beltrutti
Chronic Pain Service, Istituti Clinici Humanitas,
Rozzano (MI), Italy
Italian School of Pain Medicine (SIMED), Italy

The spinal canal is a passageway that extends from the *foramen magnum*, at the topmost boundary, to the sacrum at the lowest level. Posteriorly, it is bordered by the yellow ligament *(ligamentum flavum)* and the periosteum, and anteriorly from the posterior longitudinal ligament that lies on the dorsal part of the vertebral bodies and intervertebral discs.

The yellow ligament is a flexible structure that spans the dorsal vertebral arches of the posterior articular processes and supports the conjugate foramen. The amplitude of the spinal canal is approximately twice the width of the medulla.

The channel is wider in the cervical and lumbar regions corresponding to the swelling of the spinal cord. From C4 to C6, it measures 18 mm in the antero-posterior direction while transversely it measures 30 mm. The thoracic canal measures 17 mm in both the transverse and antero-posterior directions. In contrast, the lumbar canal is 23 mm antero-posteriorly, and 18 mm transversely. In a cross-section the channel has a triangular shape in the cervical and lumbar regions, whereas at the thoracic level the shape is more rounded.

The spinal cord at the top is continuous with the brain, while below it ends in the *conus medullaris*, at approximately the lower edge of the L1 vertebra. The dural sac contains the spinal cord and *conus medullaris*, descending to the level of S2.

The *"cauda equina"* consists of the fiber cone terminals that extend into the dural sac from L1 to S2. In the fetus, the spinal cord descends to the coccyx, but with growth, it is pushed up, due to increased growth of the spine. It follows that at birth the medulla extends only to the level of L3.

Bending of the column results in a momentary cephalad displacement of the medulla. When the nerves cannot move freely, as in the case of arachnoiditis or in the presence of fibrosis at the expense of the epidural space, excruciating pain can result.

The epidural space surrounds the dural sac, and is bounded posteriorly by the *ligamentum flavum* and *periosteum*, and anteriorly by the posterior longitudinal ligament. Laterally it is bounded by the vertebral pedicles and by the 48 intervertebral foramens. The upper limit (cephalad) of the epidural space is the *foramen magnum*, and the lower limit is the caudal end of the dural sac at S2. Technically, the sacral canal is not part of the epidural space because it does not contain the dural sac.

The posterior epidural space has somewhat different dimensions. It measures 2 mm at the cervical level, 3 to 5 mm at the thoracic level, and 4 to 6 mm at the lumbar spine. The epidural space narrows considerably between L4 and S2. The anterior epidural space is narrower, not exceeding one millimeter at any level of the column. The epidural space is rich in its content. On the medial plane, there is usually a median band of connective tissue that can be complete or may have a "cobweb-like" appearance, posteriorly connecting the *dura* to the *periosteum*.

Various anatomical structures run through the epidural space including the internal vertebral venous plexus, branches of spinal segmental arteries, lymph vessels, and the dura-arachnoid projections that surround the spinal nerve roots. There is also an abundance of adipose tissue, but the amount of epidural fat does appear to be related to the percent of body fat in an individual. The fat tissue is mainly located next to the vertebral venous plexus and forms perfect padding for the structures of the spinal cord.

The *dura mater* is a tough mantle rich in fibrous tissue with elastic fibers on the inside that cover and entirely encase the medulla. It is composed primarily of connective tissue with the fibers arranged longitudinally and a small and proportionate amount of elastic tissue. The spinal *dura mater* extends from the foramen magnum, to which it is closely adherent to the outer surface, down to the level of S2, where it ends blindly in the dura. Below this level is the "filum terminale" which follows the coccyx, where it merges with the periosteum.

Anatomical and spinal endoscopists have recommended use of the paramedian approach, and this is often used to perform lumbar epidural blocks because the vessels are concentrated at the median level.

Although spinal endoscopy may theoretically be performed at all levels of the spine, the caudal approach is recommended and is the most widely accepted method. Spinal endoscopy limited to the lumbar area is the simplest and certainly the safest. A clear understanding of the anatomy and function of the sacral canal and its content is essential for safely performing spinal endoscopy.

Some endoscopists, taking advantage of the length of certain endoscopes, tend to overcome the edge of L2. We believe that L2 represents a limit that must be respected. In our opinion SE above L2 can only be justified by proven clinical reasons and a great experience.

Sacrum - The sacrum is a bone consisting of five vertebrae fused together and having a dorsal convexity. It is located between the two iliac wings and is articulated at the top with the last lumbar vertebrae and caudally to the coccyx. On the concave front face there are four pairs of foramina that give passage to the front of the four branches of sacral nerves below. The posterior sacral foramina are smaller than their anterior counterparts. The presence of sacrospinal and multifidus muscles can prevent the spread of drugs injected into the sacral canal. On both sides of the sacral hiatus are located the rudimentary residues of the inferior articular processes which project downwards. These bony projections are called "sacral horns" and represent important landmarks for percutaneous access to the sacral canal.

It should be noted that, at the sacral level, there are significant anatomical differences determined by gender and by environmental factors, and these differences may be of considerable importance for success of the sacral epidural block.

Coccyx - The coccygeal triangle consists of three or five rudimentary vertebrae. The upper surface of the coccyx is articulated with the lower surface of the sacrum. The tip of the coccyx and the sacral hiatus together with the "sacral horns" are important landmarks when running a sacral epidural block.

Sacral hiatus – It is formed by the incomplete median fusion of the posterior elements of the lower portion of S4 and S5. This space is U-shaped and is covered in the back by the sacrococcygeal ligament, which is another important landmark for sacral epidural block. The penetration of the ligament results in direct access to the epidural space of the sacral canal.

Sacral canal – It is the natural continuation of the lower lumbar canal ending at the sacral hiatus. The volume of the sacral canal, stripped of all its contents, is roughly equivalent to 27 ml. At this level anesthesiologists and pain physicians are used to perform sacral epidural blocks. This procedure consists in the injection through the sacral hiatus of small volumes of local anesthetic (usually 5 to 10 ml) in the treatment of chronic pain or for regional anesthesia.

Contents of the sacral canal - The five sacral roots and all coccygeal nerves go through the spinal canal in the anatomical structure known as the *filum terminale*. The branches of the anterior and posterior roots from S1 to S4 come out of their respective sacral foramina. The root of S5 and coccygeal nerves leave the sacral canal through the sacral hiatus. These nerves enervate the sensory and motor nerves of their respective dermatomes and myomeres. Moreover, they also provide the innervation of various pelvic organs including the uterus, fallopian tubes, bladder and prostate.

The sacral canal also contains the sacral epidural venous plexus, which usually ends at S4, but that may go lower. Many of these vessels are concentrated at the front of the channel.

Both the dural sac and the vessels may be subject to trauma by needles, epidural catheters and spinal endoscopes. The rest of the channel is filled with fat that is subject to a proportional increase in density with age, and it has been suggested that this change could be responsible, in adult patients, for the increased incidence of the "leopard spot-shaped stain" during anesthesia for sacral epidural block.

Chapter 5

Epiduroscopic Diagnosis

Diego Beltrutti
Chronic Pain Service, Istituti Clinici Humanitas,
Rozzano (MI), Italy
Italian School of Pain Medicine (SIMED), Italy

Endoscopy of the spinal canal allows a direct view of the anatomical structures present in the epidural space such as the dura mater, yellow ligament, segmental nerves, connective tissue, fat tissue, and vessels.

This is particularly important in those clinical situations where it is difficult to reach a clear and unequivocal diagnosis. It is those cases of chronic pain in which information coming from the anamnesis and clinical evaluation of the patient does not coincide with the findings of neurophysiological tests (EMG, SSEP) and imaging (CT and MRI).

In these cases the possibility of exploring the anterior and lateral epidural space, the foramen, and the posterior epidural space can help to confirm or amend a previous diagnosis.

The transition from normal anatomy to pathological anatomy is documented by direct visualization and digital recording of the images. SE non only helps in defining a clinical diagnosis but allows for subsequent education and forensic storage. Moreover, the possibility of introducing biopsy forceps through the "working channel" allows tissue sampling from suspicious areas.

Histological examination of tissues can then confirm the diagnosis made on the basis of visual information and /or clinical examination. We can thus establish, in terms of histology, the existence of fibrosis against a nerve root or a chronic state of inflammation. More rarely is also possible to perform a biopsy on a suspected cancerous tissue.

Via the "working channel" of an endoscope there is also the possibility of introducing a dedicated spinal catheter (such as Versa-Kath® manufactured by Epimed International) in order perform lysis of the epidural adhesions according to the method of Racz or to administer local anesthetics and steroids in a targeted manner.

The precise insertion of a SCS electrode is another option that can be performed through spinal endoscopy.

In: Manual of Spinal Endoscopy
Editor: Diego Beltrutti

ISBN: 978-1-62257-250-2
© 2012 Nova Science Publishers, Inc.

Chapter 6

The Fibrosis of the Epidural Space

Lorenzo Pasquariello
SSD Pain Medicine, Ospedale Regionale U.Parini, Aosta, Italy
Italian School of Pain Medicine (SIMED), Italy

The term "epidural fibrosis" refers to all those clinical conditions where the appearance of scars or any other fibrotic tissue in some way restricts the epidural space and encompasses nerves and nerve roots. This event generally leads to the onset of nociceptive and neuropathic pain.

We can not speak of epidural fibrosis, without remembering the Failed Back Surgery Syndrome (FBSS), a painful syndrome that occurs in many people who, for different reasons, have received back surgery to remove an herniated disc, recalibrate a narrow spinal canal for congenital or acquired pathologies, or for a spinal fusion.

This post surgical syndrome, as the name itself points out, in some way expresses an opinion on whether or not the patient should be operated. In fact it is well to remember that in the United States about 1,100,000 patients each year undergo surgery on the spine. Unfortunately 40% of these patients do not get the expected result and therefore they continue to live with severe low back chronic pain.

It is possible to imagine that, in some cases, the surgical indications have been somewhat forced by the neurosurgeon or orthopedist with the intent to permanently solve the recurrent problem of a severe sciatica secondary to a disc protrusion, vertebral instability, degenerative spondylolisthesis. However it is also true that in most cases, although a careful patient selection, a correct diagnosis and despite a perfectly executed back surgery, the pain often returns after a few months.

We can not charge the sole responsibility of these painful post-operative complications to the surgery of the spine. Indeed, they can occasionally be the result of infections or arachnoiditis associated with procedures such as discography, administration of epidural corticosteroids, insertion of catheters or leads. In other words all the procedures which may have resulted in an epidural bleeding can be cause of epidural fibrosis. The medical literature also reports a case of epidural fibrosis following percutaneous disc decompression (PDD).

The postsurgical scarring or inflammation of the meninges (epiduritis or arachnoiditis) can produce patchy neurological findings difficult to interpret; in many cases MRI does not reveal specific problems. Sometimes the same neurophysiological tests can not pose a precise diagnosis.

As we have already pointed out, the epidural fibrosis has been involved as a cause of persistent pain after surgery. This issue is important not only in terms of pain and suffering but also for the economic consequences related to the state of disability and for the subsequent treatment of these persistent post surgical consequences. Besides the causes of FBSS are various and numerous. It is believed that spine surgery for spinal stenosis or herniated disc is responsible for 14.5% of cases of FBSS.

Fibrosis and adhesions in the epidural space are a normal response to surgery and can be found in the majority of patients who received back surgery. Since the formation of epidural adhesions is also found in patients who respond well to surgery, the role of lumbar epidural fibrosis in the post-laminectomy syndrome is controversial.

However, epidural fibrosis is considered to be the main cause of this syndrome by most researchers. Many surgical techniques have been proposed to minimize the formation of these adhesions. The diagnosis of epidural fibrosis after back surgery is often obtained by conventional imaging techniques such as CT or MRI, but these techniques can not detect the presence and extent of epidural adhesions in an accurate manner.

The investigation of the epidural cavity with a flexible endoscope is a new minimally invasive interventional procedure that allows the pain physician to study the epidural space with a minimal impact on the anatomical structures. In a recent study, Heavner and Bosscher, proposed the following classification of fibrosis:

Grade 1: Loose strings and sheets of fibrosis
Grade 2: More organized, continuous strings and sheets of fibrous material, non giving resistance to the endoscope
Grade 3: Dense continuous fibrous material, the endoscope can only be advanced with difficulty
Grade 4: Dense continuous fibrous material, the endoscope cannot be advanced

This classification is based in part on the degree of resistance to the progression of the instrument. Usually the flexible spinal endoscope easily passes through the epidural space and the intervertebral foramen. The presence of thick adhesions (third or fourth degree) usually prevents the advancement of the instrument. A study carried out with these criteria has enabled to classify the presence of a severe fibrosis in 83% of patients. In these people, who previously received several surgeries, it was possible to show a complete obstruction of the posterior epidural space.

We believe that spinal endoscopy should be considered an important tool in the diagnosis of epidural fibrosis. Certainly the technique requires a learning curve, but then the images of epidural fibrosis are easily recognizable.

On the other hand peridurography allows us to highlight the presence of a gap filling caused by peridural adhesions but does not allow us to diagnose an epidural fibrosis. The presence of epidural fibrosis after spinal surgery is currently diagnosed by MRI with gadolinium. With MRI, the incidence of postoperative fibrosis has been estimated in 16.7% of cases but if we consider also the severe fibrosis, it will reach 22% of cases. Spinal endoscopy not only allows us to see the presence of adhesions, but also to assess the extent of the epidural fibrosis, which is particularly useful in areas previously subjected to surgical treatment. In most patients the epidural space is completely closed. This leads to lose the communication between the upper and lower portion of the epidural space. In other words the epidural space becomes partitioned. Moreover, the compression of the dura mater, nerves and nerve roots can cause pain and neurological dysfunctions. In addition, epidural fibrosis and scarring can cause disorders in both venous and arterial local circulation.

6.1. Arachnoiditis and Pain

Clearly the fibrosis of the epidural space can accompany an adhesive arachnoiditis. The combination of mechanical and chemical factors on epidural and sub arachnoid structures brings to a complex, broad and progressive sequence of events that are capable to induce a chronic spinal pain syndrome.

It seems that many physical and chemical factors come into play in the genesis of arachnoiditis and the resulting pain. Of course nerve roots or DGG may be compressed. The results of compression are different depending upon the level of pressure exerted and upon the nerve structure involved. In rats the irritation of the DRG generates thermal hyperalgesia; hypoxia further increased sensitivity to mechanical stimuli and even provoked spontaneous firing.

The presence of scar tissue is generally associated with the loss of mobility and nerve sliding which increases its susceptibility to tension or compression. Kuslich et al. demonstrated that sciatica can be produced by stimulation of a compressed a swollen and stretched nerve root. Today it is clear that the DRG and not the dorsal roots are responsible of the pathological response to compression since DRG are highly sensitive to local increase in pressure.

While high pressure can damage the integrity of the nerve structure, low pressure usually produces an impaired blood supply, resulting in a nerve edema, reduced nutritional transport which can lead fibrosis. It has been demonstrated that an epidural pressure equal to arterial blood pressure stops the blood supply to the cauda equina. When a pressure of 10 mm Hg is applied the result is a 20-30% reduction in nutrient transport to nerve roots. This altered circulatory situation can determine an impaired supply of oxygen to nervous structures within the affected area.

Compression and scar presence in the sub arachnoid space can also lead to disturbances in the CSF flow which may cause local but also distant effects that are expressed in the dilation of the thecal sac. Alterations in the CSF circulation could account for unexplained upper body symptoms in patients who have lumbosacral arachnoiditis in the absence of pathology in thoracic or cervical regions.

Referring to the action of inflammatory substances it is clear that peripheral nerve endings become sensitised by chemical mediators released during tissue damage and inflammation such as substance P, bradykinin, histamine and prostaglandins. Also chemical irritants that originate in the nucleus pulposus (material from an herniated disc) are held accountable for the genesis of persistent spinal pain. Protoglicans, suc as IL-1, IFN and TNF-alpha are more or less neurotoxic.

As a result, loss of input from impaired nerves and damaged DRG may trigger a compensatory upregulation of central receptors. This situation open the way to a central sensitisation.

In conclusion we can say that epidural fibrosis, sometimes in combination with arachnoiditis is a real clinical problem for patients who did undergo spine surgery. Imaging we get from CT and MRI do not really highlight the challenges that are present and that can be evaluated only by direct vision of the epidural space.

In: Manual of Spinal Endoscopy
Editor: Diego Beltrutti

ISBN: 978-1-62257-250-2
© 2012 Nova Science Publishers, Inc.

Chapter 7

Patient Evaluation

Diego Beltrutti
Chronic Pain Service, Istituti Clinici Humanitas,
Rozzano (MI), Italy
Italian School of Pain Medicine (SIMED), Italy

Prior to the procedure of spinal endoscopy, patients will be evaluated by a pain clinician. The specialist will perform a complete clinical examination to clearly define the patient's neurological status.

Since spinal endoscopy is reserved for complex cases of chronic or persistent pain in the spine, there is a need for providing an accurate history, results of recent pre-intervention tests, a blood coagulation profile, and spinal column imaging tests such as X-ray, dynamic radiographs of the spine, CT, or MRI. A complete clinical work-up may also include a comprehensive physical examination performed by a pain clinician with additional consultations by specialists in orthopedics, physiatry, neurosurgery, neuropsychiatry, or psychology.

Among the tests often considered necessary in the preoperative phase are Electromiography (EMG), Quantitative Sensory Testing (QST), nerve conduction velocity (NCV), Somato Sensorial Evoked Potentials (SSEP).

Before providing a final clinical opinion, the clinician should correlate results of imaging studies with the findings of neurophysiological tests and those that emerge from the physical evaluation. For the purpose of diagnosing sacral low back pain, dynamic X-rays may be useful when they are performed with the spinal column in flexion, extension and in an oblique position, especially for those cases where we must better define or exclude pathological conditions that would not benefit from performing spinal endoscopy.

MRI examination has become indispensable in cases of chronic low-back pain. Radiologists can usually provide a thorough explanation of the images. However, it is also important that the pain clinician understands how to read the MRI, specifically looking for problems of spinal stenosis, bulging disc, and lesions of the articular processes in order to evaluate the anatomical relationship between those structures in the spinal canal that may be generating pain.

Once proposed, the suggestion of performing spinal endoscopy should be carefully reviewed to insure that there are no conditions present in the patient that may constitute an absolute or relative contraindication. All conditions are then reported in the medical records. The medical file also needs to include the patient's informed consent to the procedure, which must be obtained after a clear and simple explanation of the objectives of the procedure and including the mild and serious complications as well the prognosis and risks of not performing the procedure.

7.1. Pharmacotherapy

NSAIDs, aspirin, and anticoagulants should be discontinued at least five days before the procedure. The mode of interruption of aspirin and antiplatelet therapy obviously varies with the type of cardio circulatory disease of the patient. Clinicians have to consider if there is a risk of bleeding or risk of thrombosis. In this regard it is advisable to follow the leading guidelines and recommendations of scientific societies in terms of administration and discontinuation of antiplatelet drugs.

The clinician should consider the need for therapy with subcutaneous low molecular weight heparins (LMWH). The coagulation profile of the patient should be assessed (partial thromboplastin time, INR, and platelet count).

Usually the bleeding associated with spinal endoscopy is limited and occurs distally at the sheath at the sacral hiatus. Regarding the use of other drugs (anti hypertensives, cardiotonics, diuretics, etc.), the patient can safely continue to take his/her basic therapy.

We remember that opioids are not among the drugs to be discontinued before a pain procedure. When the pain experience is severe, opioids must be used.

7.2. Analgesia, Sedation and Monitoring

After obtaining written consent from a patient for implementation of spinal endoscopy, the pain clinician should reassess the patient in a subsequent visit and the results of preoperative tests requested and re-evaluated. At this time, the pain clinician will also need to explain to the patient the type of monitoring that will be used, the pre-anesthesia protocol, and the arrangements with the anesthesiologist for the level of analgesia.

The clinician should explain the reason that the procedure cannot take place under general anesthesia, but must be done using local anaesthesia and analgesia. The need for maintaining voice contact during the entire procedure should be explained and emphasized to the patient, so that it is clear to the patient that the clinician can be constantly and immediately informed of the state of consciousness of the patient and any changes that may occur.

Local anesthesia is performed at the entry point to the sacral level. To improve patient comfort during the procedure, administration of intravenous fentanyl (50-100 μg) can be used. Deep sedation should be avoided because the patient must be conscious and able to communicate with the clinician during the procedure.

In the case of particularly anxious subjects, which happens quite often, pre-medication with a short-acting hypnotic drug such as intravenous midazolam (0.015 mg - 0.03 mg/kg IV) is recommended. This drug does not interfere heavily with the state of consciousness and does not induce prolonged recovery time.

Patient monitoring must include non-invasive blood pressure (NIBP), peripheral oxygen saturation (oximetry or SpO2), and ECG. The patient should have venous access and an anesthesiologist must be present or immediately available to manage any eventuality that may arise during the procedure.

7.3. Preparation of the Patient

The evening before the procedure the patient should take a shower, carefully and thoroughly cleaning the lumbar and sacral areas. It is recommended fasting from solid foods and liquids (milk, fruit juice) at least six hours and clear liquids (water, tea, chamomile) for at least three hours. In the case of anxious patients, it is recommend that they take 1 mg Lorazepam sublingually the night before the surgery.

7.4. Preoperative Preparation

The morning of the intervention, the operating room personnel should check the availability of the necessary equipment and material for the procedure, from the connections to the functioning of the column for video laparoscopic surgery. The presence of a suitable fluoroscope (digital dual screen is recommended) and the availability of the radiologist technician should be confirmed. Remember to check that the operating table have a radiotransparent floor.

During this phase, we suggest that the clinical folder should be carefully checked by the operator for the patient's consent to the procedure, which should also provide information on the technique as well as its potential risks. Ideally, the patient should have signed the consent form at least seven days before surgery in order to allow the patient time for reflection and to request further explanations of the procedure and its benefits and risks.

Under no conditions should it be considered appropriate to have the consent form signed by the patient while on the operating table.

The Centre's staff will have to confirm, before the acceptance of the patient for intervention, the availability of a bed for "one-day surgery." The patient arrives from home on the morning of the intervention but then he will spend one night at the hospital. It is neither safe nor recommended that a patient be sent home immediately after spinal endoscopy. Even in the case of diagnostic SE.

7.5. Sterility

Spinal endoscopy is performed in the operating room under strict hygienic conditions and procedures that maintain absolute sterility. Although it is a percutaneous procedure, the clinician, after thorough and careful disinfection of the hands, should wear a sterile gown, sterile gloves, hat and mask. We also recommend the use of leaded eyewear to reduce the risk of eye damage.

Under the gown, the clinician must wear a leaded jacket and a dosimeter for measuring absorbed radiation since fluoroscopy is used during procedure.

Thirty to sixty minutes before the beginning of the procedure, the patient should receive an intravenous antibiotic as prophylaxis. This prophylaxis usually consists of a single dose, and among the more frequently used antibiotics are ceftriaxone (1-2 gr. IV), cefuroxime (1.5 gr. IV), and ciprofloxacin (150 mg. IV).

7.6. Patient Positioning on the Operating Table

The position of the patient should be prone, with arms stretched forward, resting on the armlets, with the forearms slightly bent 90° downwards. It is advisable to place a pillow under the abdomen to align the spine, with placement of another pillow under the back of the feet so that toes do not touch the bed. This creates a more comfortable position for the patient.

The operating table must be positioned for maximum maneuverability of the fluoroscope, and it is important to have a completely radiotransparent operating table. The patient should be fully monitored (NIBP, HF, SpO_2, ECG). An intravenous infusion needle (18 gauge) should be inserted into the right arm. The patient is admitted for "one-day surgery" in the case of diagnostic endoscopy, or for a minimum stay of about two days when it is associated with lysis of epidural adhesions in accordance with the procedure of Racz.

Even when spinal endoscopy (SE) is used only for diagnostic purposes it is advisable that the patient spends one night in hospital in order to be discharged the next day. The patient receives antibiotic therapy (e.g. ciprofloxacin or similar at a dose of 1-2 g/day IV) about thirty minutes before procedure, hydration therapy by intravenous infusion of Ringer's solution, and analgesics. We are used to start with an initial dose of 50 micrograms of IV Fentanyl as a routine. This dose can be increased later if necessary.

Sedatives should be avoided because the patient must be conscious and able to communicate with the clinician during the procedure.

In: Manual of Spinal Endoscopy
Editor: Diego Beltrutti

ISBN: 978-1-62257-250-2
© 2012 Nova Science Publishers, Inc.

Chapter 8

Indications

Diego Beltrutti

Chronic Pain Service, Istituti Clinici Humanitas,
Rozzano (MI), Italy
Italian School of Pain Medicine (SIMED), Italy

The main indications for spinal endoscopy are related to those cases where it becomes important to have direct visualization of the epidural space. Therefore, from a diagnostic point of view, spinal endoscopy becomes important in the presence of radicular pain without a clearly identifiable pathology of the intervertebral disc. Many of the patients have nerve roots encapsulated with adhesive scar tissue, clinical inflammatory changes and traction on the nerve root.

The diagnostic indications include young patients suffering from unexplained sciatica (radicular pain due to radiculopathy or radiculitis) devoid of surgical indications and who have not responded to conservative therapy; spinal endoscopy may distinguish pathologies that are also different from the syndrome of radicular compression.

In many cases where there is radicular pain in the absence of pathology showing root compression, spinal endoscopy has enabled visualization of the presence of an inflammatory condition that may be caused by the action of endogenous chemical irritants. To explain the shared bio-humoral factors of inflammation result in these painful conditions in the presence of negative or weakly positive CT and MRI findings, it has even been suggested a "leaky disc." It has been possible to identify specific pathologies on the affected roots including fibrous lacineae, adhesions, neuritis, and yellow ligament hypertrophy.

8.1. Patient Selection

During the selection of patients for spinal endoscopy, the clinician must remember that the observed symptoms can be related to biochemical problems (e.g. root irritation due to chemical, toxic, vascular, or degenerative components) as well as anatomical problems (e.g. narrow channel, space-occupying lesions, scars, fibrosis, etc.). When determining whether this procedure is appropriate for a particular patient, both the symptoms and anatomical variables should be considered. Symptoms that potentially represent a state of radiculopathy and that likely arise from multiple causes may respond positively to the direct administration of saline, local anesthetics, or steroids.

The chemical mediators responsible for inflammation-immunity can result from a herniated *nucleus pulposus* or synovial facet tissue as well as other sources. These irritants may act in combination with canal stenosis, fibrous adhesions and cysts in producing radiculopathies.

Symptoms that may favorably predispose to a procedure of spinal endoscopy include disorders referable to lumbar and sacral radiculopathies, neuralgias, and plexopathy from the irritation of nerve roots in the absence of significant compressive lesions.

Since elderly patients often present a stenosis of the spinal canal, we recommend to perform spinal endoscopy in young people, under the age of 60. Moreover we recommend always that spinal endoscopy be preceded by sacral peridurography. In this way it will be possible to realize the location of the epidural fibrosis within the epidural space, the extent of the adhesions to be destroyed and the limitations of movement of the endoscope.

The presence of a compressive lesion, with conspicuous signs of progressive neurological impairment, constitutes a contraindication, at least relative, for further injection of fluid in the epidural space. The medical literature provides evidence that the best clinical results occur when spinal endoscopy was used in a specific subgroup of patients. This subgroup was characterized by acute and subacute spinal pain attributable to disc pathology in the absence of learned pain behaviours and without undergoing spinal surgery.

It is likely that this subgroup responds positively to a "washout" of chemical irritants and to the anti-inflammatory effect of steroids. These patients would not be characterized by neuroplastic changes in the CNS. The lack of a framework for neuroplasticity and secondary hyperalgesia would be a determining factor for a positive response to treatment only for the "washout" technique. Endoscopy of the spinal canal is not recommended in patients with pain syndromes such as myofascial syndromes or those based on biomechanics such as facet syndrome or sacral iliac joint dysfunction.

8.2. Indications of Spinal Endoscopy

Indications of spinal endoscopy can be divided into those of the diagnostic and therapeutic types. The strength of its diagnostic use is the ability of direct visualization of the epidural space in those complex cases where there is no evident correlation with what has been shown by imaging tests (X-ray, CT, MRI, etc.), neurophysiological tests (e.g. EMG, SSEP), symptoms reported by the patient, and evidence obtained by physical examination.

According to recommendations available in medical literature, spinal endoscopic adhesiolysis seems to be an effective treatment modality for chronic refractory low back pain and radiculopathy that is related to epidural adhesions.

Therapeutic indications for spinal endoscopy include those analgesic techniques that take advantage of the opportunity to have a direct view of epidural space structures, thereby allowing precise administration of drugs (such as in adhesiolysis), or precise allocation of specific devices in well defined areas of the epidural space (such as in SCS electrode positioning).

Spinal endoscopy demonstrates that the prevalence of severe epidural fibrosis after back surgery is substantially higher than is generally reported in MRI evaluations. Today it is clearly accepted that severe fibrosis and thick adhesions in the epidural space constitute an underlying pathology in most patients with FBSS.

Currently accepted indications:

- diagnostic improvement in complex spinal pain syndromes of unclear etiology
- persistent unexplained radiculopathy without surgical indications and when there is lack of response to conservative treatment
- targeted positioning of epidural catheters and targeted chemical lysis of adhesions related to FBSS
- implantation of electrodes for neurostimulation (SCS) in the epidural space in technically difficult cases

- mechanical lysis under direct vision of adhesions and fibrous scar tissue adherent to anatomical structures at the epidural level (nerve roots)
- biopsy of tissues present in the epidural space
- visual support for minimally invasive pain procedure

Probable indications:

- puncture and aspiration of epidural cysts (Tarlov cysts)

Now let's see a little more in detail the different indications:

- *Diagnostic improvement in complex spinal pain syndromes of unclear etiology.* The technique can "visually" analyze the anatomical structures present in the epidural space. This is particularly useful when information of clinical and imaging (e.g. CT, MRI) are conflicting.
- *Persistent unexplained radiculopathy without surgical indications and when there is lack of response to conservative treatment.* Spinal endoscopy offers the opportunity for various types of interventions in painful pathologies of different spinal origins. This can be done through targeted administration of analgesic solutions (e.g. local anesthetics and steroids), through a combined pharmacological and mechanical action (e.g. by the Racz procedure, injection of a targeted hypertonic saline solution, local anesthetics, and hyaluronidase) or by the application of laser or radio frequency systems (e.g., lesion of adhesions using RF or laser energy).
- *Targeted positioning of epidural catheters and targeted chemical lysis of adhesions related to FBSS.* The targeted positioning of epidural catheters such as Versa-Kath® or similar devices can be used to precisely administer steroids and analgesic solutions. In FBSS, steroids are often injected via epidural into areas of least resistance, which often are the areas where there is no pathology. With spinal endoscopy under fluoroscopic control it is possible to accurately administer the drugs, thus optimizing the therapeutic mechanisms.
- *Implantation of electrodes for neurostimulation (SCS) in the epidural space in technically difficult cases.* Today the technique of spinal cord stimulation (SCS) is spreading in a range of old and new directions.

The need to position the electrocatheter in specific areas can be achieved by inserting the electrode under direct visualization during spinal endoscopy.

- *Mechanical lysis under direct vision of adhesions and fibrous scar tissue adherent to anatomical structures at the epidural level (nerve roots).* Lysis of adhesions can be obtained with different modalities. It can be done through mechanical action, pharmacologic techniques, use of laser or RF. It is obvious that the mechanical action of a flexible spinal endoscope is very different from and superior to the mechanical action of an epidural catheter.
- *Visual support for minimally invasive pain procedure.* There have been reports in the literature of video-assisted procedures to approach the spinal cord avoiding the use of contrast medium as well as vascular injuries and consequent unpredictable neurological deficits. Spinal endoscopy can provide an useful visual aid in complex cases of vertebroplasty, disc decompression, cervical antero-lateral cordotomies, trigeminal nucleo-tractotomies and selective rhizotomies.
- *Biopsy of tissues present in the epidural space.* There are several clinical conditions for which a epidural biopsy can be used to make or to confirm a diagnosis. One of the advantages of spinal endoscopy is to use the endoscope's working channel into which a biopsy forceps can be introduced, thereby enabling a sample to be obtained that can be used to histologically document what was previously seen on CT or MRI.
- *Puncture and aspiration of epidural cysts.* About this indication there is still no consensus among clinicians. However there have been reports in the literature of clinicians who were able to drain these cysts by insertion of the tip of the spinal endoscope.

The ideal candidate for spinal endoscopy should have a health-oriented lifestyle; possibly be still working; have no medico-legal problems; be taking minimal medication with no behaviors indicative of the potential for addiction; and an absence of secondary gains.

The best pain relief is obtained in young people, who have not been submitted to surgical procedures on the back and with MRI which reveals a limited presence of fibrous tissue.

8.3. Complex Cases of Spinal Pain

The patient with chronic spinal pain often presents a complex picture. While symptoms and clinical presentation may be clearly related to the spinal column, these disorders are often in conflict with the results of diagnostic imaging. Moreover, these patients have frequently already undergone spinal surgery. In these cases, endoscopy of the spinal canal can potentially be used to define the presence, location and clinical relevance of:

- spinal nerve root compression
- scars resulting from spinal surgery
- internal fixation
- different pathologies into the epidural space
- epidural adhesions
- stenosis of the spinal canal

Although there is not always a clear cause/effect relationship in chronic pain, the possibility to exclude or confirm situations of potential or actual lumbar pain constitutes a major therapeutic potential of spinal endoscopy.

Current FDA approved indications for SE are:

- documentation of decompression structures
- documentation of pathological aspects in the spine
- direct inspection of nerve and nerve roots
- direct inspection of internal fixation
- precise delivery of therapeutic agents in the epidural space.

In: Manual of Spinal Endoscopy
Editor: Diego Beltrutti

ISBN: 978-1-62257-250-2
© 2012 Nova Science Publishers, Inc.

Chapter 9

Key Aspects of the Technique

Diego Beltrutti
Chronic Pain Service, Istituti Clinici Humanitas,
Rozzano (MI), Italy
Italian School of Pain Medicine (SIMED), Italy

About thirty minutes before the procedure, the patient should be given antibiotic prophylaxis intravenously, as we have already recommended in chapter 7.5.

Since the use of fluoroscopy is indispensable for the procedure, the clinician must wear a lead apron under the sterile gown, as well as a thyroid protector and a dosimeter to measure absorbed radiation. Using a pair of "x ray" glasses is highly recommended for those who often use fluoroscopy.

The patient is positioned on the operating table in the prone decubitus position, taking care to maintain the patient's comfort. A patient who is not comfortable tends to move and increases the difficulty of the procedure. It is useful to have the patient's legs slightly bent back by placing a foam pad at the ankles.

If the patient has a pronounced lordosis, a radiotransparent pillow can be placed under the abdomen, positioned between the operating table and the anterior iliac crest in order to minimize the lordosis of the lumbar vertebral column. After thorough disinfection of the skin with antiseptic solutions (two washes with iodopovidone solution for surgical use and one of chlorhexidine), the sterile surgical field should be prepared using 4 sheets of nonwoven tissue or a specific drape for spinal endoscopy. The fluoroscope should be covered with two sterile disposable covers for the "C" arm.

As already mentioned, the clinician should wear a hat and surgical mask and, after adequate surgical scrub of the hands, put on sterile gloves and a sterile gown.

Identification of the sacral hiatus should be performed in the standard manner (palpation of the sacral horns), and identification of the sacral canal will require a fluoroscopic radiogram using a latero-lateral view, with subsequent penetration of the skin overlying the sacral hiatus and the sacrococcygeal ligament.

The clinician initiates the procedure by inserting a cutaneous bolus of local anesthesia (3-5 ml of lidocaine 2%) with a short 25 gauge needle. Then, using a 22 gauge needle applied to the wheal already raised by the bolus of anesthesia, the deeper layers are infiltrated with 1% ropivacaine, providing a more prolonged analgesia.

The tip of the needle can be used for palpation in order to better assess the position of the sacral hiatus. At this point, a 1 cm skin incision should be made with a scalpel "blade 11" to dissect the coccygeal ligament covering the sacral hiatus. This maneuver facilitates the subsequent insertion of the dilators and cannula. The edges of the incision can be slightly expanded using a surgical instrument such as a small Kelly forceps.

A 17 or 18 gauge epidural needle[1], such as is inserted through the incision into the sacral canal. The correct position of the needle can be assessed by fluoroscopy in AP projection if the clinician needs to direct the needle toward the right or left, but especially laterally.

If the position seems to be correct, a contrasting agent such as amipaque sodium can be injected. Usually, 2 - 3 ml of a water-soluble nonionic contrast medium will be sufficient to resolve all doubt. The injection of a contrast agent is also useful to assess compliance in the distension of the epidural space. If there is little compliance, the contrast agent will go up very high in the canal. In the case of good compliance, it will rise one or two vertebrae at most. This maneuver is very useful because the presence of poor compliance at the time

---

[1] We use and suggest epidural needles such as the flexible Introducer Cannula (SCA) over a 17 GA Tuohy needle. This introducer, that is a radiopaque low friction (fluoropolymer) sheath, is shear resistant providing fault free catheter access and manipulation into the epidural space. This is a definite advantage for operators who are in the acquisition phase of the technique. For more expert clinicians we suggest the RX coudé epidural needle. These needles are produced by Epimed Int. USA.

of injection of the physiological saline will increase awareness of the potential for onset of high intra-epidural pressure with its inherent risks.

If the channel is well injected, the Seldinger technique can be used to introduce a wire guide through a specific epidural needle, as we mentioned above. It should be moved forward up to L5-S1 by carrying out numerous fluoroscopic controls during the maneuver in order to follow its progression in the sacral canal.

The guidewire is preferably directed into the anterior side of the epidural space, a position that better enables visualization of foramina and roots. Inexperienced endoscopists sometimes insert the instrument into the posterior of the epidural space, in which case spinal endoscopy will give poor results because this position is not at the more appropriate level of the foramina.

At this point, the dilator is ready to be inserted with the assistance of the metal guidewire. The clinician's experience will help get it through the hiatus into the sacral canal by a gentle exertion of circular movements left and right and associated with slight pressure in order to preserve the internal integrity while encouraging ascension into the canal.

This first dilator (12 Fr diameter) is sent forward over the guide wire and is inserted in order to reach the sacral canal. When the clinician can feel that it has entered and is moving well in the right channel by gliding freely on the guidewire, the dilator can be removed. At this point, a second dilator (9Fr) is introduced into sacral canal, on which the introducer is mounted.

If the dilator and the introducer move well in the canal, the dilator and guidewire can be drawn back while leaving the introducer inserted. At this point the targeted video guide for spinal endoscopy is inserted through the cannula that should now be correctly positioned in the sacral canal.

A 0.9% saline solution (normal saline) is administered through the side channel of the video guide in amounts from 1 to 10 ml in order to wash away debris or clots that can impair endoscopic visualization, as well as to lubricate the sliding channel of the endoscope.

In order to facilitate viewing and maintain sterile washing of the video circuit, the authors suggest to use a 500 ml bag of saline placed in a "squeeze-bag" system with a constant pressure of 40 mm Hg. This methodology allows quick charging of the 10 ml Luer-Lock syringe and, at the same time, keeps closed the washing circuit preventing from external accidental contamination.

While the procedure of spinal endoscopy requires specific technical steps, there may be some differences depending on the material and equipment that is used. The procedure described here is related to the use of the EPI-C (Equip Medikey). The choice of this spinal endoscope is dictated by the conviction of the authors that this equipment is one among the most advanced among those presently available. This is mainly due to the presence of the lens mounted on the tip of the video guide which does not require the use of a sterilized optic fiber.

Subsequently, an optical fiber 0.9 mm (10,000 pixels) in diameter is inserted into the video guide through a dedicated channel. The use of a greater number of pixels would be certainly beneficial for the purposes of vision, however, the problem is that an increase of pixels also leads to an increase in the diameter of the optic fiber. The presence of a larger diameter makes quite difficult the insertion of the fiberscope through the sacral canal.

The second channel of the video guide is connected to the washing circuit. As we mentioned before, the use of a fixed and pre determined pressure exerted by the squeeze bag should prevent from excessive spikes of pressure into the epidural space. In case the operator needs more pressure it can be increased in a sterile manner by using, with caution, the 10 ml syringe as a valve.

Before insertion into the sacrum, the clinician must balance the white, adjust the focus of the camera and understand the direction of the camera's movement. It is recommended that writing be used for verification by matching, so that the writing on top corresponds with the top of the image, and the bottom writing with the bottom of the image. Without this help, the clinician can be convinced of going in one direction when in fact the movement is in another direction.

After making these maneuvers, the clinician should introduce the video guide in the sacral channel through the previously inserted cannula.

Under direct endoscopic control, and with absolute caution, the pain clinician directs the video guide in a cephalic direction by making it progress through the epidural channel moving it in an antero-lateral direction.

The clinician should use lateral fluoroscopy to verify that the instrument is located at the antero-lateral position and subsequently in AP to evaluate the side and location of the apex of the instrument. The saline can be used for irrigation by applying pressure for brief periods and in small quantities to help distend the epidural space so that it exceeds the focal length that allows clearer visualization.

However, care must be used for the administration of saline to avoid prolonged excessive pressure in the epidural space that could seriously compromise perfusion of the neural structures.

Authors agree that a maximum volume of 100 ml should be used, and it is thought that this volume is sufficient to complete the procedure safely. The proteolytic enzyme hyaluronidase (900 IU) can be added in order to facilitate dissection of adhesions or inflammatory scars. Additionally, at the end of the procedure and under direct visualization, the steroid triamcinolone (40 mg) can be administered through the endoscope. Some spinal endoscopists are also used to inject 150 micrograms of clonidine in combination with 8 ml ropivacaine 0.2% at the end of the procedure. The low concentration of local anesthetic is chosen in order not to interfere with motor activity.

As already mentioned, the administration of saline enables constant and optimal viewing of the endoscopic surgical field and at the same time allows washing. It is important to check that the taps on the base of the working channel are open so that they can function as a safety valve for the epidural space thus preventing excessive pressure reaching the channel.

Currently, techniques are being developed to measure the pressure within the epidural space in order to avoid the excess pressure that could lead to significant neurological *sequelae* (consequences).

The procedure is performed under local anesthesia so that the patient can promptly report the onset of a nuchal headache, which is a sign of excess pressure within the spinal canal.

It should be noted that through the "working channel" much of the injected saline will be displaced when the channel is occupied by small instruments such as a biopsy forceps. It is useful to collect this amount in a bag to assess the actual volume in the channel, which provides an estimate of the difference between the quantity injected and how much of it has been displaced.

Under direct viewing, it will also be possible to evaluate the patient's response resulting from the mild and gentle touch, performed by the tip of the instrument, of the afflicted nerve roots: an accurate expression of the pain that normally affects the patient would most precisely indicate the source of the pain itself.

We want to stress the fact that spinal endoscopy provides needs accurate and gentle maneuvers as excessive force, and rapid movements increase the likelihood of complications.

The Italian company Policare has developed a stimulation catheter (Stim-Cath®) that enables stimulation, under direct visualization, of the root suspected as the source of pain using an electronic stimulator similar to those used for the localization of the plexus in regional anesthesia. This is another useful aid to the definition of spinal pain generators. In this way it is possible to assess whether the pain we have caused through nerve stimulation is consistent with the pain that patient usually feels.

If it is decided that there is a need to perform mechanical lysis of adhesions present in the epidural space under direct endoscopic view, peridurography should be done before starting the lysis procedure. A radiogram can be obtained by positioning the fluoroscope in LL and AP in order to document the initial situation. The mechanical lysis of the adhesions can then be accomplished under visual monitoring through the gentle movement of the tip of the instrument.

Generally, the passage of the video guide itself is able to open a gap large enough to allow communication between the upper and lower anterior epidural space. If the gap is not considered large enough, through the working channel it is possible to place an epidural catheter designed for adhesiolysis[2] according to the method of Racz.

The use of a laser source or molecular quantum resonance radiofrequency are additional methods that may be effective for removal of adhesions, although certainly more risky. These therapeutic modalities are reserved for a small sphere of pain clinicians with a long experience as these energy sources can easily give rise to complications if not used with great care.

Fluoroscopic imaging is used to monitor the segmental level at which the instrument is operated. In the past, some endoscopists have tried to dilate the epidural space and break adhesions with the use of a Fogarthy catheter.

The use of Fogarthy's balloon is no longer recommended because the balloon easily breaks and it is possible that the resulting fragments remain in the epidural space causing a foreign body inflammatory reaction.

Some spinal endoscopists are used to perform a peridurogram at the end of the procedure using 5 ml of contrast medium (amipaque sodium 300) in order to evaluate the outcome in terms of resolution of the stenosis (assessed by differences in filling of the spinal canal and intervertebral foramen by the contrast agent). Currently this practice has been abandoned in order not to produce a further dilution of the injected drugs.

Before removing the video guide, 50 mg epidural Ciprofloxacin can be administered as antibiotic prophylaxis, and after removal, the sacral incision is closed with the application of a silk suture, and a medicated gauze is applied.

The procedure for spinal endoscopy cannot be performed as an outpatient (ambulatory surgery) or day case surgery procedure (same day in and out), but must be done with as ODS or hospitalization, with at least one night spend as an inpatient. The amount of time spent in hospital depends on the

---

[2] For this purpose we suggest a catheter like Versa-Kath® (from Epimed int., USA) or Stim-Cath® (from Policare, Italy).

organizational system or on the guidelines of the pain centre. We usually discharge the patient the day after the procedure, after a complete rest in the supine position for 24 hours. Upon discharge, the patients in provided with a letter containing recommendations and information regarding post-surgical therapy.

In: Manual of Spinal Endoscopy
Editor: Diego Beltrutti

ISBN: 978-1-62257-250-2
© 2012 Nova Science Publishers, Inc.

Chapter 10

Recognizing Endoscopic Images

Attilio Di Donato
Anaesthesia and Pain Medicine Service,
Ospedale Concordia per Chirurgie Speciali, Roma, Italy
Italian School of Pain Medicine (SIMED), Italy

Recognition of the appearance of various anatomical structures in the spinal canal, and in particular those located within the epidural space, is crucial for diagnosis and for maintaining orientation during the procedure. Equally fundamental is the simultaneous use of fluoroscopy, since it enables the clinician to know the position of the video guide at any time in the different areas of the epidural space (anterior epidural space, posterior, antero-lateral or postero-lateral, left or right). Fluoroscopy is also useful for informing the clinician of the level reached by the tip of the endoscope.

In the event that there is no sense of direction within the channel, it is very likely that the instrument will be advanced in the posterior epidural space rather than in the antero-lateral direction that allows access to root pockets. In this case, using a simple fluoroscopic latero-lateral projection, it can be confirmed whether or not the endoscope is correctly inserted into the epidural space. Besides the ability to recognize structures such as the dura, yellow ligament, nerve roots, and blood vessels, it is necessary for the clinician to memorize the structures and images the comprise the anatomical formations present at the subarachnoid level. The prompt recognition of these structures will allow the clinician to immediately confirm the passage of the instrument from the epidural space to the subarachnoid space. In this case it will be possible to immediately interrupt a procedure that accidentally intrudes into the subarachnoid space. One of the main indicators of this event is the absence of bleeding and high visibility of structures that are immersed in the CSF.

10.1. Planning of Spinal Endoscopy

Another point is that an endoscopy has to be carefully planned in advance. Do not confuse an endoscopic procedure with an interesting photographic tour up and down the epidural space. The patient arrives at the operating table after being thoroughly evaluated and provided with an admission diagnosis and/or a suspected disease or alleged pathology defined on the basis of clinical evaluation and imaging. It will be toward this diagnosis that the clinician should direct their attention and the spinal endoscope. In this way the spinal endoscopy will be a diagnostic aid and not a photographic "safari" *in corpore vili (*latin term to indicate a *worthless body)*.

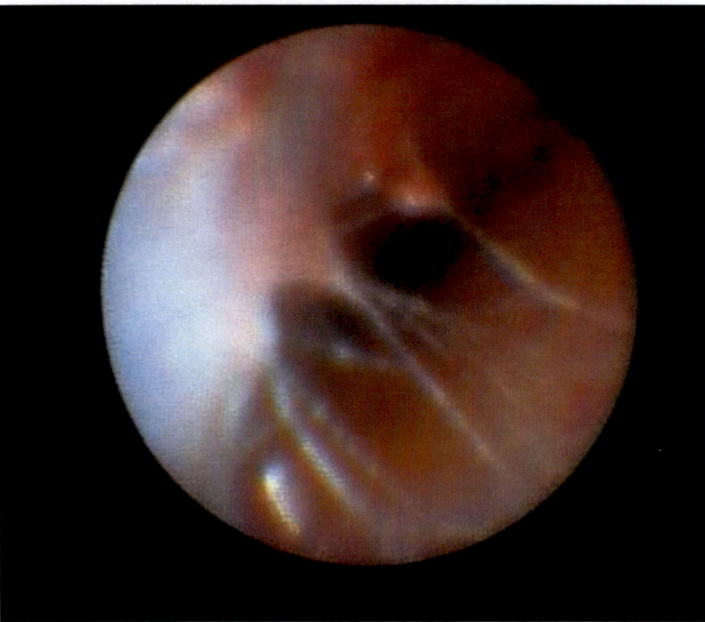

Figure 10.1. Some fibrous adhesions coming from *dura mater* that limit the amplitude of the epidural space. Bright red colours show the presence of a big inflammation. The tissues are tinted and edematous.

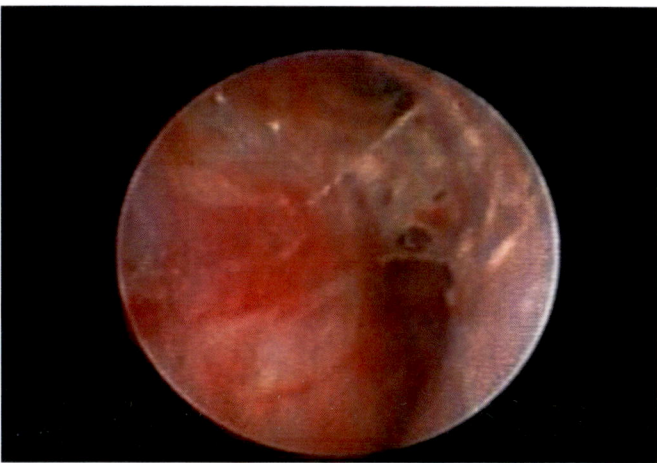

Figure 10.2. Signs of inflammation in the epidural space with dropdown adhesions.

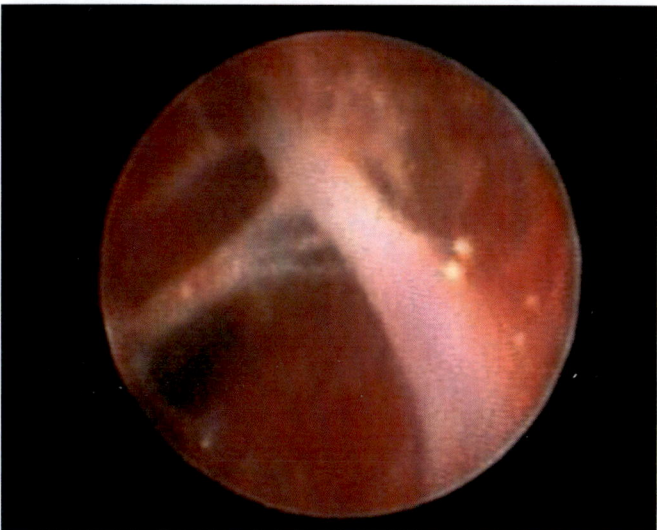

Figure 10.3. Nerve root crossing the epidural space that looks hyperemic, swollen with fibrotic adhesions that limit its mobility.

We suggest to use a timer. Spinal endoscopy should be completed within a maximum duration of 30-40 minutes. Defining and agreeing on the timing of the procedure with the patient will make it more easily tolerated. A quick procedure means injecting a smaller amount of saline, a reduced risk of traumatic effects, and a reduced risk of severe complications.

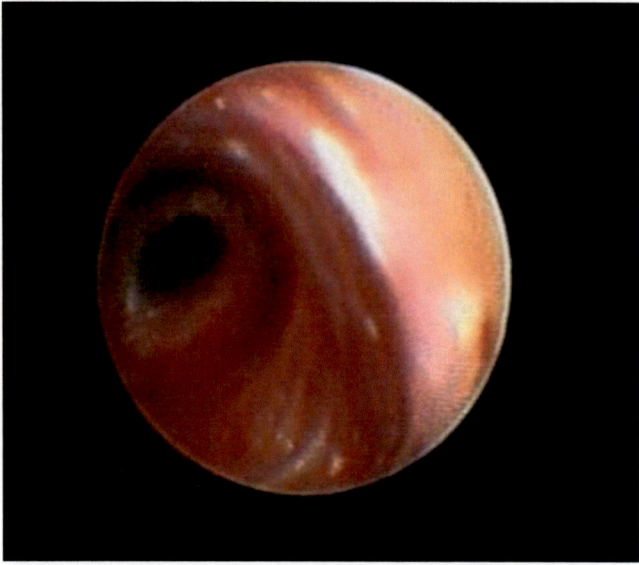

Figure 10.4. Patent and stenotic epidural space with fibrin deposition which suggests a chronic inflammatory state. The tissues are hyperemic, swollen, edematous with signs of fibrosis.

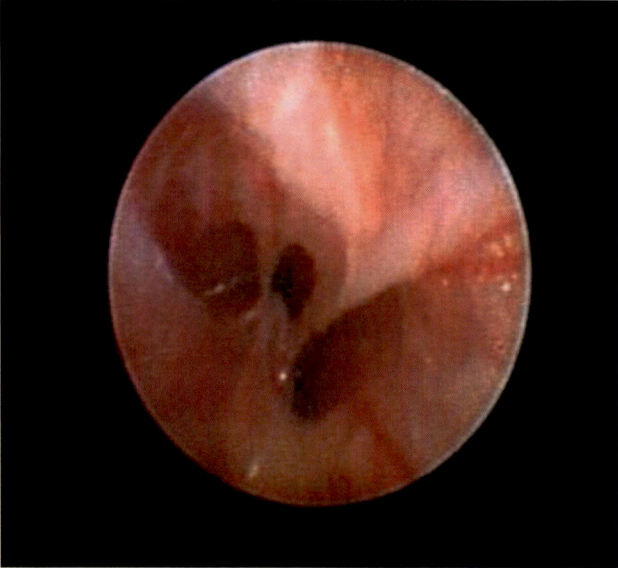

Figure 10.5. The visual field shows a plica in the epidural space. Fibrous adhesions and septa are present. The area is crossed by a nerve root.

The medical literature suggests an endoscopic procedure with no set time limits and that continues "ad libitum" is associated with a greater risk of neurologic complications from direct or secondary trauma and to increased hydrostatic pressure inside the spinal canal.

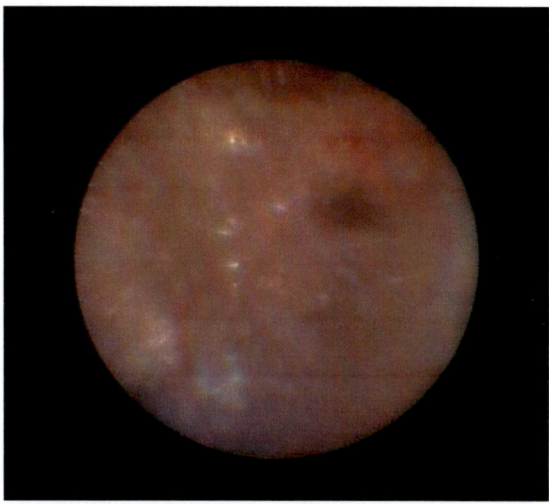

Figure 10.6. Epidural fat covering the *dura mater*.

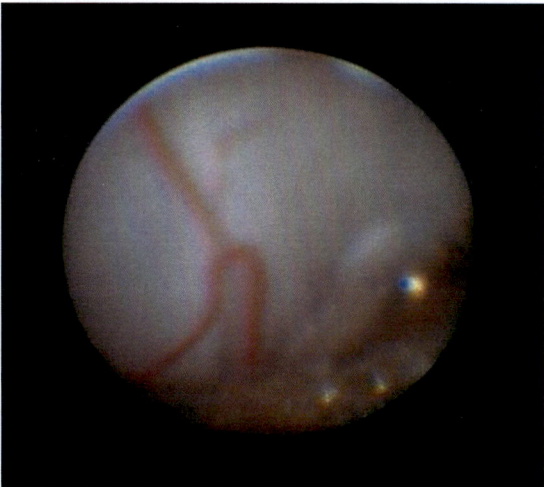

Figure 10.7. The *dura mater* shows its typical pearly appearance. The visual field is crossed by some venous capillaries. Right and below we note the presence of epidural fat.

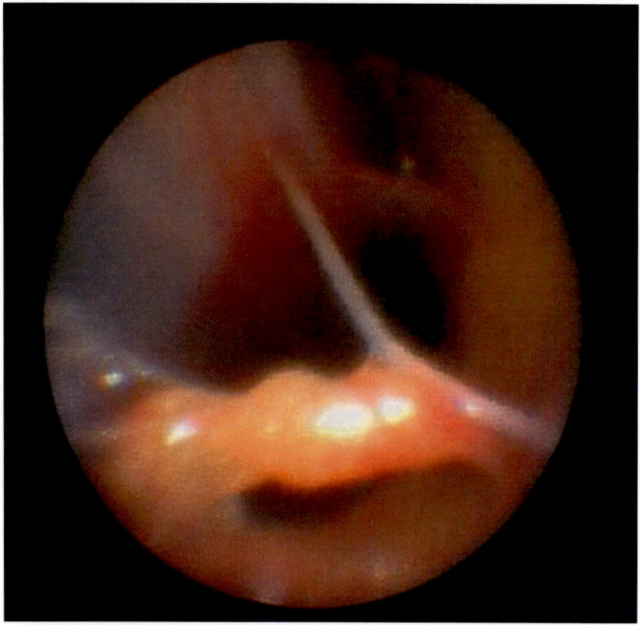

Figure 10.8. Fatty septum with a small fibrotic adhesion; on the left is possible to see the *dura mater* with some fibrotic adhesions.

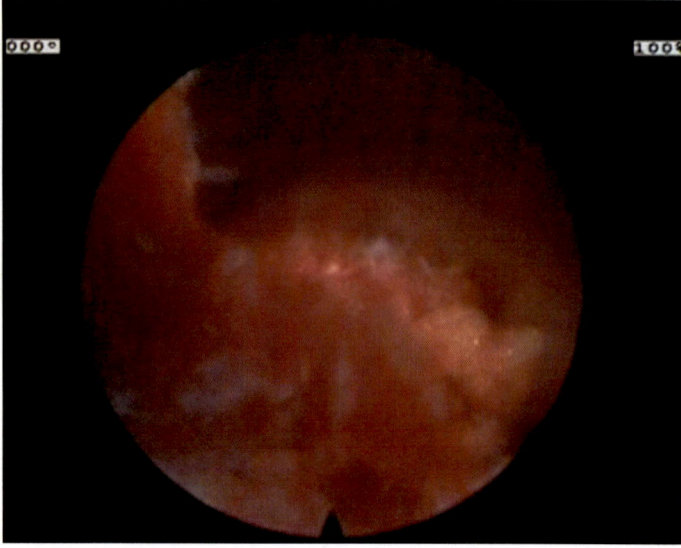

Figure 10.9. The whole visual field is occupied by inflammatory scar tissue.

Here are some images of the endoscopic epidural space. In the absence of an atlas of images and other forms of training useful for the recognition of normal or pathological epidural structures, we have included some representative images that we hope will help young people who come to this technique by allowing them to more easily recognize some anatomical structures.

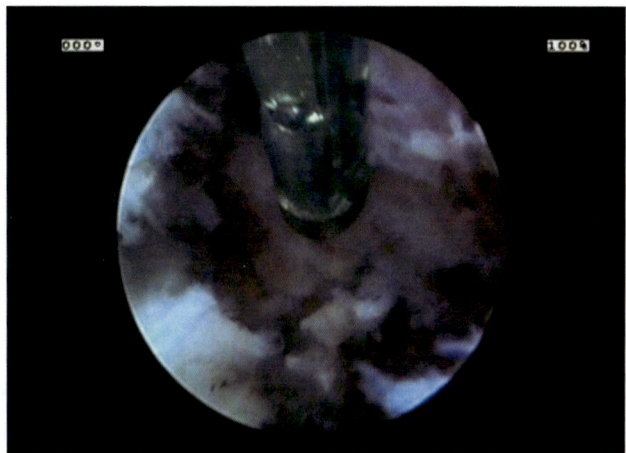

Figure 10.10. In the top center, in green : tip of the RF device working to free the L5 root.

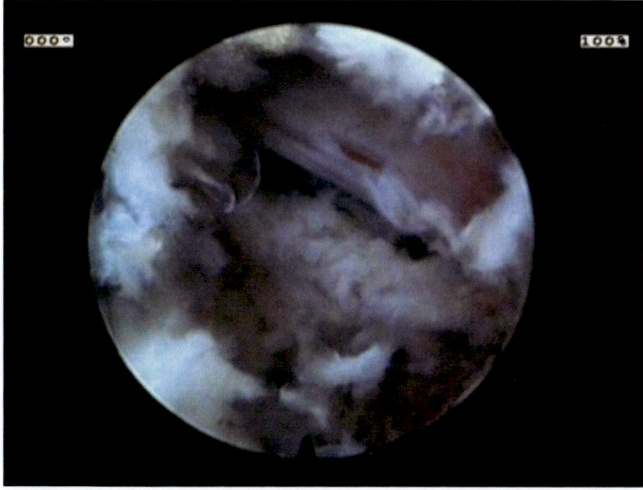

Figure 10.11. After reclamation of the scar tissue inflammation the L5 root (top) is free and mobile from fibrous scar along its course.

Chapter 11

After the Procedure

Diego Beltrutti
Chronic Pain Service, Istituti Clinici Humanitas,
Rozzano (MI), Italy
Italian School of Pain Medicine (SIMED), Italy

Following the procedure, having given one or two stitches, medicated gauze will be applied at the caudal level to cover and aseptically isolate the area where the Tuohy needle, the cannula and the endoscope were inserted.

At this point, the patient is taken from the operating room to the recovery room, where the patient will remain at rest, lying down, for about two hours for observation before being sent to the ward. A nurse will monitor the heart rate and blood pressure, and peripheral oxygen saturation is measured using a blood oximeter, which is a transcutaneous sensor applied to a finger. The intravenous infusion cannula will be maintained up to discharge from hospital.

At the end of the procedure the pain physician will prepare the report on the procedure performed. This documentation, together with a copy of the medical record and instructions for the first days after surgery, should be delivered by the patient to their general practitioner.

This medical documentation should contain not only a clinical description of the procedure but also a summary of the diagnosis and details of any therapy provided. The duration of the procedure, amount of saline used, and the type and amount of antibiotic injected after the procedure should also be stated as part of the medical record.

After the procedure and before discharge, the patient should undergo a neurological examination. Any new neurological deficits should be evaluated carefully and seriously. In case of doubt concerning the possible occurrence of a serious neurological complication, the clinician should promptly carry out an imaging exam (MRI, CT) and provide the patient with a neurological or neurosurgical consultation.

It is important to give the patient detailed hygiene instructions and emphasize their importance. These instructions consist of the method for perineal cleaning after defecation, which should be directed from behind forwards, so as not to involve the area subjected to the endoscopic procedure.

Patients should be advised not to bathe for five days, and although a shower is permitted starting from the third day, it should be fast rather than of prolonged duration.

11.1. At the Time of Discharge

After a hospitalization of at least one night, the patient can be discharged provided that the neurological examination is normal and there is no bleeding or other complications; a guide or driver should accompany the patient home. Upon reaching home, the patient should be supervised by a friend or a family member throughout the immediate post-intervention period.

As sometimes a troublesome and persistent pain can be present in the sacral region for some days that may even be of moderate to severe intensity, the use of oxycodone 5 mg orally 1-2 times per day may be useful. When an NSAID is to be used, we administer ibuprofen arginine salt 600 mg/day. Patients who were already on oral opioids before spinal endoscopy will have to continue the same doses as before. Only later it will be possible to evaluate the opportunity to start a program of weaning from opioids.

The oral administration of anti platelets anti thrombotitic agents has to be discontinued before procedure in order to reduce the risk of bleeding. If there is a need to reduce thromboembolic risk, the use of LMWH or unfractioned heparins is recommended.

As mentioned previously, antibiotic therapy and an oral anti-inflammatory should be administered for about 5 days. After seven days, it will be possible to remove the sutures, and three days after that the dressing may be removed.

Regarding physical activity, it is suggested that the days following the procedure should be considered a period of active rest at home, only resuming those light daily activities that are considered essential. Driving or operating machinery is not recommended during the first 24 hours after discharge. It should be remembered that it is very important to protect the entry point where the endoscope was inserted into the sacral hiatus with a dressing to prevent bacterial contamination. If the dressing should come off, the entry point should immediately be disinfected and a new dressing applied.

In: Manual of Spinal Endoscopy
Editor: Diego Beltrutti

ISBN: 978-1-62257-250-2
© 2012 Nova Science Publishers, Inc.

Chapter 12

Maintaining Sterility

Diego Beltrutti
Chronic Pain Service, Istituti Clinici Humanitas,
Rozzano (MI), Italy
Italian School of Pain Medicine (SIMED), Italy

Almost all materials used for the performance of endoscopic spinal procedures are sterile and disposable including dilators, cannulae, and the video guide. However, the fiber optic system is not disposable, and dependent on the video guide that is being used, adequate sterilization may be required with each use.

12.1. "Adequate Sterilization" of Neurosurgical Equipment

There are some endoscopes used for spinal endoscopy (like the Myelotec video guide) that have an open tip through which the optic fiber comes in direct contact with the epidural tissues and the fluids that are present. Other endoscopes do not have this possibility since the optic fiber is located in a working channel completely closed distally by a lens. This is the case of EPI-C Equip Medikey video guide. Thus, adequate sterilization of neurosurgical instruments means that the optic fiber coming into contact with nerve tissue should be sterilized using techniques that can destroy not only bacteria but also prions.

12.2. The Prions

The word "prion" is derived from its English description of being an "only proteic infectious particle". The term is an acronym derived from proteinaceous infectious only particle. This name was given to these unconventional infectious agents that consist exclusively of proteins and are apparently devoid of nucleic acids.

Isolation and characterization of prions were a result of research by the American scientist Stanley B. Prusiner, and this discovery earned him the 1982 Nobel Prize for Medicine. Prions are the infectious agents responsible for the group of diseases known as spongiform encephalopathies, which include bovine spongiform encephalopathy (mad cow disease), scrapie in sheep, and Creutzfeldt-Jakob disease (CJD) in humans. These degenerative nerve diseases are characterized by the presence of groups of intensely vacuolated neurons in certain brain areas that give the brain a spongy appearance, and of "Alzheimer's type" amyloid plaques with the absence of any inflammatory reaction.

These pathogenic agents, that are transmissible, are able to induce abnormal folding of specific normal cellular proteins called prion proteins that are found most abundantly in the brain. The functions of these normal prion proteins are still not completely understood. The abnormal folding of the prion proteins leads to brain damage and the characteristic signs and symptoms of the disease. Prion diseases are usually rapidly progressive and always fatal (CDC data).

The prion is composed of proteins conjugated to sugar moieties (sialoglycoproteins). However, infectious prions are extremely resistant to the degradative effects of most chemical, physical, and biological agents common used for procedures of disinfection and sterilization including proteases, heat, and formalin treatment.

In the absence of nucleic acid material (DNA or RNA), scientists believe that the replicative cycle of prions, so far unique in nature, is based on a biochemical mechanism whereby an infectious prion interacts with prion proteins normally contained in animal cells. The "bad" prion induces changes in normal protein conformation and molecular structure, converting these normal proteins into pathogenic prion particles. Therefore, the prion is neither a bacterium nor a virus, but rather a simple protein with unique characteristics.

12.3. The Need of an Accurate Sterilization of Neurosurgical Equipment

Data from CDC confirm that iatrogenic transmission of the CJD agent has been reported in over 250 patients worldwide. These cases have been linked to the use of contaminated human growth hormone, dura mater and corneal grafts, or neurosurgical equipment. Of the six cases linked to the use of contaminated equipment, four were associated with neurosurgical instruments, and two with stereotactic EEG depth electrodes.

All of these equipment-related cases occurred before the routine implementation of sterilization procedures currently used in health care facilities. No such cases have been reported since 1976, and no iatrogenic CJD cases associated with exposure to the CJD agent from surfaces such as floors, walls, or countertops have been identified.

12.4. The Creutzfeldt-Jakob Disease (CJD)

According to CDC, Creutzfeldt-Jakob disease (CJD) is a rapidly progressive, invariably fatal neurodegenerative disorder believed to be caused by an abnormal isoform of a cellular glycoprotein known as the prion protein. CJD occurs worldwide and the estimated annual incidence in many countries, including the United States, has been reported to be about one case per million population.

The vast majority of CJD patients usually die within 1 year of illness onset. CJD is classified as a transmissible spongiform encephalopathy (TSE) along with other prion diseases that occur in humans and animals. In about 85% of patients, CJD occurs as a sporadic disease with no recognizable pattern of transmission. A smaller proportion of patients (5 to 15%) develop CJD because of inherited mutations of the prion protein gene. These inherited forms include Gerstmann-Straussler-Scheinker syndrome and fatal familial insomnia.

Creutzfeldt-Jakob disease (CJD) and its variant (vCJD) are rare human diseases, although it cannot be excluded that human-to-human transmission can occur due to contaminated instruments used in surgery. Consequently, in order to protect the population against all pathogenic forms of CJD, international regulations have been developed that require a mandatory sterilization process for all instruments that come into contact with the nervous system or its components.

12.5. Sterilization Methods Outlined in Annex III of the WHO Infection Control Guidelines for Transmissible Spongiform Encephalopathies

Effective sterilization for reducing the risk of infection with surgical instruments that come in contact with nervous structures is essential. The three most stringent sterilization methods for heat-resistant instruments described in Annex III of the WHO guidelines are listed below; the methods are listed in order of more to less severe treatments. Sodium hypochlorite may be corrosive to some instruments. Before instruments are immersed in sodium hypochlorite, the instrument manufacturer should be consulted about the instrument's tolerance of exposure to sodium hypochlorite. Instruments should be decontaminated by a combination of the chemical and recommended autoclaving methods before subjecting them to cleaning in a washer cycle and routine sterilization (CDC data).

1. Immerse in a pan containing 1N sodium hydroxide (NaOH) and heat in a gravity displacement autoclave at 121°C for 30 min; clean; rinse in water; and subject to routine sterilization[1].
2. Immerse in 1N NaOH or sodium hypochlorite (20,000 ppm available chlorine) for 1 hour; transfer instruments to water; heat in a gravity

---

[1] CDC Note: The pan containing sodium hydroxide should be covered, and care should be taken to avoid sodium hydroxide spills in the autoclave. To avoid autoclave exposure to gaseous sodium hydroxide condensing on the lid of the container, the use of containers with a rim and lid designed for condensation to collect and drip back into the pan is recommended. Persons who use this procedure should be cautious in handling hot sodium hydroxide solution (post-autoclave) and in avoiding potential exposure to gaseous sodium hydroxide, exercise caution during all sterilization steps, and allow the autoclave, instruments, and solutions to cool down before removal.

displacement autoclave at 121°C for 1 hour; clean; and subject to routine sterilization.
3. Immerse in 1N NaOH or sodium hypochlorite (20,000 ppm available chlorine) for 1 hour; remove and rinse in water, and then transfer to open pan and heat in a gravity displacement (121°C) or porous load (134°C) autoclave for 1 hour; clean; and subject to routine sterilization.

12.6. Problems Connected to the Use of Open Tip Spinal Endoscopes

Going back to our optical fiber, a Pain Center using Myelotec video guides must have several optical fibers available. The need for frequent sterilization will lead to rapid deterioration of the fibers, resulting in reductions in resolution and image quality. Therefore, despite the substantial costs associated with acquisition of these fibers, there is a necessity for changing them frequently and early, before image quality is compromised.

The situation is different for the EPI-C Equip Medikey video guide or similar close tip spinal endoscopes, since in this video guide, because of the closed tip, the optical fiber is not exposed to epidural fluids. Moreover the optic fiber cannot leave the video guide because the channel is sealed at the tip by the presence of a lens. Thus, in this spinal endoscope, the optical fiber does not come into contact with either nerve tissue or surrounding fluid in the epidural space. This fact is very important because not being forced to sterilize the optical fiber it will prolong life, maintaining at the same time the visual properties of the endoscope.

One of the advantages of the EPI-C Equip Medikey video guide is that it is not necessary to sterilize the optical fiber, which translates into lower utilization costs. In fact a Pain Center will not need to buy or rent multiple optical fibers. Moreover, by not having to sterilize the optical fiber, it can be used for at least twice the number of procedures before showing signs of wear, thereby providing greater savings and practicality of use.

In: Manual of Spinal Endoscopy
Editor: Diego Beltrutti
ISBN: 978-1-62257-250-2
© 2012 Nova Science Publishers, Inc.

Chapter 13

Contraindications

Attilio Di Donato
Anaesthesia and Pain Medicine Service,
Ospedale Concordia per Chirurgie Speciali, Roma, Italy
Italian School of Pain Medicine (SIMED), Italy

Spinal endoscopy is a minimally invasive percutaneous technique, and as such is characterized by a low level of morbidity. Nevertheless, there are clinical situations and conditions that contraindicate its use. Since the technique involves inserting a probe (flexible fiberscope or endoscope) into the epidural space through a small incision at the sacral hiatus, contraindications to this procedure are similar to those of epidural anesthesia. These contraindications are divided into those that are absolute and those that are relative.

13.1. Absolute Contraindications

- Cerebral vascular diseases
- Deficits of the central and/or peripheral nervous system in a non-stabilized phase
- Epilepsy, including even a remote history of episodes
- General anesthesia
- Inability to maintain a prone position

- Inadequate equipment
- Inadequate training of the operator
- Lack of consensus
- Malformations of the spinal column and/or sacrum
- Pregnancy
- Presence of septic lesions
- Previous brain surgery
- Renal and/or hepatic insufficiency
- Serious coagulopathies
- Severe respiratory insufficiency
- Unstable angina, CHF.

13.2. Relative Contraindications

- Chronic persistent headache
- Concurrent presence of many and diverse painful disorders
- Ongoing and untreated psychiatric disturbances
- Retinal diseases, partial blindness
- Severe stenosis with or without myelopathy
- Somatoform disorders
- Unrealistic expectations

The procedure of spinal endoscopy is accompanied by the need to inject a certain volume of saline, which can result in the creation of high pressure within the epidural space. Additionally, the actual introduction of the flexible endoscope into the epidural space can lead to mechanical and traumatic effects. In both of these cases, side effects may occur. Based on these considerations, as we already pointed out in the list of absolute contraindications, it should be noted that the procedure must be avoided in those patients with:

1. Unwilling to consent or an inability to give valid consent to the procedure. The consent of the patient must be expressed in a valid way. We recommend using an *ad hoc* form to obtain consent.
2. Major malformations of the sacrum that may prevent the introduction of the epidural needle and accessories (e.g. absence of the sacral hiatus, presence of pilonidal cysts, stenosis of the sacral canal, etc.).

3. Septic and dystrophic skin lesions at the sacral hiatus such as anal fistulas, osteomyelitis of the sacrum, etc. If there is a risk of contaminating the canal and the epidural space with potentially infective material, with the possibility of causing meningitis or meningismus, the procedure should be delayed until the situation is resolved.
4. Spinal cord abnormalities: meningeal cysts, meningomyelocele (spina bifida).
5. Inability to maintain the prone position for at least 60 minutes (COPD, CHF, unstable angina, etc.). During the procedure the patient is awake and cooperative in order to insure comprehensive monitoring of the local and general neurological conditions. It is not advisable to try to perform spinal endoscopy on a patient who is moving or is intolerant of the required position. Once all appropriate measures are adopted to ensure comfort in the prone position, such as use of gel-filled cushions at the points of decubitus, and the analgesia protocols have been initiated, the operation should nevertheless be stopped if the patient becomes non-cooperative. In some cases, the potential for patient non-cooperation can be foreseen and avoided beforehand.
6. Pregnancy.
7. Renal insufficiency.
8. Severe respiratory failure (severe chronic obstructive respiratory diseases such as COPD).
9. General anesthesia. The occurrence of narcosis does not necessarily indicate that the clinician can recognize at an early stage serious complications such as epidural bleeding with compression at the level of cauda.
10. Chronic hepatic insufficiency.
11. History of bleeding in the stomach and/or bowel. A patient who is at risk of bleeding should not be considered a candidate for spinal endoscopy.
12. Coagulation abnormalities. For patients with coagulation abnormalities, available guidelines should be followed, such as those of the European Society of Regional Anaesthesia and Pain Therapy (ESRA).
13. Clinical situations characterized by an actual or potential increase in intracranial pressure (ICP), e.g. primary or secondary brain tumors, pseudobrain tumor, and cerebrovascular diseases. The administration of saline, both in relation to the volume of liquid used and to the

injection pressure used, can lead to changes in the intracranial pressure.
14. Presence of bladder or intestine dysfunction (cauda equina syndrome, problems of urinary dynamic, sphincter malfunctions).
15. Presence of neurological disorders such as foot drop.
16. Sexual disorders with particular reference to impotence. If there are problems with sexual function, there is a risk that future problems may be attributed to the procedure and/or to the clinician. In this case, the procedure is not recommended.
17. Toxic and infectious conditions.
18. Known allergy to drugs used in the procedure (history of adverse reactions to NSAIDs, local anesthetics, contrast agents, etc.).
19. Chronic intake and or abuse of narcotics and/or alcoholic beverages. Spinal endoscopy should be used only after a cessation program for the use of these substances.
20. Inadequate equipments (lack of availability of a video column, radiolucent operating table, digital fluoroscope with still imaging, etc.).
21. Inadequate training of the operator.

In: Manual of Spinal Endoscopy
Editor: Diego Beltrutti

ISBN: 978-1-62257-250-2
© 2012 Nova Science Publishers, Inc.

Chapter 14

Complications

Diego Beltrutti
Chronic Pain Service, Istituti Clinici Humanitas,
Rozzano (MI), Italy
Italian School of Pain Medicine (SIMED), Italy

As with all invasive procedures, complications may occur. The professional curriculum of the pain clinician, his/her experience and skill, comprehensive and accredited training, strict observance of the rules of asepsis-antisepsis, and compliance with the rules of technology including maintaining the established processing times, are all key factors that contribute to reducing the risks related to the procedure.

I remember one of my teachers in this field one day he said to me: "*At that time we were so excited about what we were looking in the spinal canal that seemed to be crazy. We were going up and down with the epiduroscope as to choose the best place to stop for a picnic. Then we started to give us a maximum time limit of thirty minutes and a to focus on a specific target* ".

Complications that may occur include:

- Incorrect positioning of the epidural needle resulting in the administration of air and drugs in subcutaneous tissue, in the sacral canal, in the sacrococcygeal ligament, in the bone cavity of the sacral vertebrae, or in the pelvic cavity

- Accidental vascular puncture and intravascular administration of local anesthetic
- Accidental injury of the *dura mater*
- Neurological deficits secondary to epidural hematoma (e.g. paresis or paralysis)
- Post dural puncture headache (PDPH)
- Transient dysesthesia
- Retinal hemorrhage or other neurological complications; these complications generally are secondary to high and sustained pressure during the saline infusion
- Pain, abnormal sensitivity and/or diffuse spasms in the legs during or immediately after the procedure; also in this case complications are related to the administration of excessive amounts of saline into the epidural space
- Urinary retention from administration of local anesthetics and/or opioids at the level of the sacral nerve roots
- Infections
- Allergic reactions.
- Pain at the surgical site.

However, these complications of spinal endoscopy are generally of two types: malposition of the needle and generation of excessive hydrostatic pressure in the epidural space.

14.1. Related to Malposition of the Needle

Side effects that may occur during or after the procedure of spinal endoscopy are similar to those found with simple caudal epidural injections. In fact, the needle may be positioned incorrectly outside the sacral canal due to difficulties in identifying the sacrococcygeal ligament or the sacral hiatus, thereby resulting in injection into subcutaneous tissue.

Another possible displacement of the needle may occur when the tip is in direct contact with the sacral periosteum. This results in substantial pain accompanied by a high resistance to the injection and an inability to administer volumes greater than a few milliliters of solution. A third cause of bad positioning is the possibility that the needle tip is within the ligament without having gone through it, and this is a determinant of resistance and pain during the injection.

Much more serious is positioning of the needle in the medullary portion of the sacral vertebra. Whenever there is a problem of injecting only a few milliliters of saline or local anesthetic, it will be necessary to monitor and control the position of the needle using fluoroscopy.

Another serious error is the introduction of the needle into the pelvic cavity through the sacrum or through a side access to the coccyx. In this case, the needle can penetrate into the rectum and/or into the vagina causing serious contamination that can lead to major infections when the needle is repositioned in the sacral canal.

The incidence of these complications related to the positioning of the needle can easily be reduced by using fluoroscopy for visualization during the stages of the procedure for introducing the needle in the sacral canal. We strongly suggest to exclude erroneous positioning of the needle with a fluoroscopical lateral view.

Since the sacral epidural space is highly vascularized, the possibility of intravascular administration of local anesthetics and/or drugs is significant and thus careful aspiration and incremental dosing of the anesthetic is required in order to monitor possible intravascular passage of the drug. In case of doubt, the infusion of a small amount (2 ml) of contrast agent such as sodium metrizamide (Amipaque) will clarify the possible intravascular insertion of the needle.

After the caudal block, the incidence of neurological deficits secondary to the epidural hematoma is rare but can nevertheless occur. Consequently, patients need to be carefully monitored both during and after the procedure.

Neurological complications are extremely rare and are usually associated with pre-existing injuries and/or to trauma due to an improper use of the technique.

As previously mentioned, the use of high infusion pressures of saline, normally the result of the infusion of large amounts of saline, may impair blood flow within neural structures present in the epidural space and therefore must be absolutely avoided. It should also be kept in mind that, although uncommon, side effects and complications may still occur especially in immune compromised patients or in those with malignancies.

14.2. Related to Generation of Excessive Hydrostatic Pressure in the Epidural Space

As previously mentioned, spinal endoscopy requires, at some point of technique, infusion of local anesthetics and analgesic mixtures into the epidural space. In order to prevent neurotoxic effects, the use of substances without preservatives is recommended, as is use of filtered solutions for injection[1].

The administration of known volumes of saline is essential as this allows the flexible fiberscope to reach its specific focal length and enable visualization of the relationships among the anatomical structures present in the epidural space.

During spinal endoscopy, it is necessary to monitor the injected fluids and keep the volume as low as possible. Total volume should not exceed 100 ml. If the patient complains of pain after the clinician has introduced a small volume of saline, this usually indicates that the epidural space has very low compliance. This is a potentially hazardous situation because it can lead to transmission of excess pressure in areas more distant from where the fluids have been administered through the CSF.

When the patient begins to complain about the onset of headache or vision disorders, the clinician should consider changing the operating plan and/or immediately terminate the procedure. Excessive epidural pressure may negatively interfere with either local perfusion at the level of spinal nerve roots, segmental nerves or the vascularity of remote areas.

The onset of pain between the shoulder blades during the procedure suggests high epidural pressure, and should result in the termination of the procedure because of concerns regarding development of retinal hemorrhage. These complications are presumably due to the transmission of pressure which has built up inside the spinal canal, potentially reaching the brain and disrupting retinal perfusion and/or resulting in macular hemorrhage.

---

[1] It is known that opening glass and/or plastic vials is associated with a problem of micro fragments. The injection of micro fragments of any material into the dura and/or epidural space may result in significant fibrosis. We recommend that Safe Shot filters (by Policare: www.policare.net) or similar devices be used as these are designed for filtration under suction and allow injection of solutions into the epidural space without the need for other procedures during injection. The clinician can thus maintain sensitivity at different stages of epidural or subarachnoid injection procedures.

The pain present in the surgical site is usually minor and self-limiting. The pain arising in different areas distant from the surgical site requires careful and prompt assessment and medical documentation. These painful conditions, including severe headache, dysesthesia and excruciating back pain, may be representative of the onset of a potentially severe complication such as an epidural hematoma, spinal ischemia, or high hydrostatic pressure. These different and dangerous clinical situations must be immediately ruled out. Paresis, paralysis and severe pain may be complications of direct trauma to neural structures caused by the passage of the epiduroscope, or can be the consequence of the presence of epidural hematoma, high hydrostatic pressures with secondary ischemic effects. Visual disturbances and blindness have also been reported. However, the incidence of these complications is rare and has been previously reported during routine performance of epidural blocks.

The appearance of local bleeding at the surgical site rarely causes neurological complications since the entry point of the cannula is just above the coccyx. While bleeding may predispose to infection, this is rare.

It should be strongly suggested to patients that they take a shower the night before the procedure, paying particular attention to washing the sacral and lumbar areas. We suggest to colleagues our protocol consisting of a thorough disinfection of the skin using iodopovidone (two times) and chlorhexidine (once) in order to achieve a sterile surgical area. Antibiotic prophylaxis should be given to the patient to reduce the risk of infectious complications.

Post-intervention, the wound should be kept dry for three days, and after defecation the anus and rectum should be thoroughly cleaned in a set pattern starting at the anus and moving forward. This point is very important in the first three days after procedure.

14.3. Persistent Headache

Persistent headache, which can be severe in intensity, is caused by leakage of the CSF subsequent to puncture of the *dura mater*. This specific headache is called PDPH or post dural puncture headache. It usually persists for several days, but rarely for a few weeks. From the literature it shows that the administration of fluids, bed rest, and utilization of NSAIDs is enough in most cases to control the symptoms. In persistent cases it may be suggested to apply an epidural blood patch with homologous blood.

14.4. Dysesthesia and Severe Lumbo-sacral Pain

These disorders may result from the presence of an epidural hematoma, spinal ischemia, or high hydrostatic pressure at the epidural level. Their presence indicates the need for neurological evaluation and clinical monitoring, and in some cases a CT or MRI may be urgently required. Although these are extremely rare situations, the clinician should always be prepared in advance to take appropriate action should these conditions arise during or after the procedure.

14.5. Retinal Hemorrhages

Retinal hemorrhages in the macula and inner layers of the eye may occur when an excessive volume of saline is injected into the epidural space, causing a rapid and sudden increase in intracranial pressure. The transmission of increased pressure inside the spinal canal upwards through a secondary increase in CSF pressure may reduce retinal perfusion or cause macular hemorrhage. This complication is potentially serious since there have been reports in the literature of persistent visual disturbances and blindness. Although the actual incidence of these events has not been determined it is probably low. This complication is possible even after epidural block.

14.6. Generation of Pain during Injection of Saline in the Epidural Canal

Excessive pressure cannot only be caused by injection of large volumes of saline, but also by injection of small amounts of saline into confined spaces. Such excess pressure may especially be generated when the presence of fibrous tissue limits the dispersal of liquids up, down, or laterally toward the foramen. At this level, in normal subjects, Sharpy fibers allow fluid to flow out into the extra dural space.

In some subjects the presence of fibrous tissue, scarring, the adhesion of the epidural space and epidural septation can prevent the proper functioning of the Sharpy fibers and create real peri radicular closed pockets. The injection of fluids in one of these bags will lead to a sudden increase in the local pressure with the following risk of ischemic damage to neural structures.

From Olmarker and Rydevik we know that cauda equina blood supply is interrupted when epidural pressure is equaling arterial blood pressure. 10mmHg applied pressure caused 20-30% reduction in nutrient transport to nerve roots.

As already mentioned, increase in pressure within the epidural space can cause perfusion problems at a local or remote level.

Patient complaints of neck or scapular pain during the procedure generally indicate that the epidural pressure has increased and the patient may be at risk for retinal hemorrhage. Additionally, complaints of pain after infusion of even a small amount of saline solution may indicate that the distensional ability of the epidural space is compromised (e.g. because of a narrow channel or septation), and the increased CSF pressure, is felt even in distant areas. The volume of saline to be injected in the epidural space must be kept low, and the clinician must constantly be in verbal contact with the patient. Only through such constant communication will the clinician be able to tell if the discomfort that the patient reports requires either a change in the procedure or its immediate termination.

14.7. Infections

After spinal endoscopy, there is a risk of infection of the subcutaneous tissue, as well as a risk of subdural infection or abscess, arachnoiditis, meningitis or meningismus. The occurrence of these infectious events may be due to several causes including the failure to follow the rules of asepsis, the use of contaminated materials, or the presence of an infectious outbreak that may not be clinically obvious. The importance of washing well at home before the procedure should be emphasized to the patient. Upon arrival at the Pain Center, the patient should receive antibiotic prophylaxis at least thirty minutes before the procedure.

In the operating room, the gluteal, sacral, and coccygeal areas should be thoroughly cleaned with surgical disinfectant, and a surgical field should be prepared using a surgical set specifically for this procedure.

At the end of the endoscopic procedure, a surgical dressing should be positioned at the entry point of the spinal endoscope at the level of sacral hiatus. This measure is usually sufficient however in some cases one or two stitches may also be required.

The patient should be instructed that, after defecation, the anal and rectal areas should be cleaned from behind forwards. The dressing should be kept dry for at least the first three days and the patient should take oral antibiotics for at least 4 days.

14.8. Direct Nerve Injury

There is a possibility of direct nerve injury. In theory, the nerves most at risk are those travelling into the sacral canal, particularly in cases of a very narrow canal. However, this risk is minimal since introduction of the instrument is done slowly and carefully, and the patient, being awake, is able to report promptly any discomfort or pain. The consequences of direct nerve injury are dependent on whether the lesion is complete or partial, and cannot only increase preexisting pain, but also lead to paralysis of muscles innervated by the specific root affected, or sensory symptoms such as paresthesia, dysesthesia, tingling, or numbness.

14.9. Paresis, Paralysis and Pain

These complications may be the result of different actions: an incorrect epidural needle passage, improper use of the Seldinger technique, or clumsy insertion of the spinal endoscope or dilator (traction, stretching, section, avulsion). They may also be associated with the presence of an epidural hematoma or an increase of hydrostatic pressure (at first in the epidural and then at the subarachnoid level). Additionally, they can occur secondary to the condition of ischemia (root, spinal cord, retina, etc.). It is stressed once again that the best therapy is prevention. A constant conversation with the patient during the procedure and great delicacy in surgical maneuvers is the best way for good results avoiding neurological complications.

14.10. Accidental Dural Puncture

Dural puncture is a rare complication that may be caused when an instrument penetrates the dura and enters the subarachnoid space. This can happen if the spinal endoscope is pushed forward in the absence of visual control. Another possibility is that the optic fiber alone advances too far beyond the cannula, although this does not occur with the EPI-C Equip Medikey endoscope since it has a closed tip. The pain physician must remember that, for open tip fiberscopes such as those made by Myelotec, it should always be possible to see a small crescent in the visual field that is formed by the edge of the cannula as seen from the optical fiber located within the cannula.

This image tells us that there are no risks that the optical fiber is out of his channel in the fiberscope. The constant presence of a small crescent in the visual field reassures us as to say that the optical fiber could not pierce the dura or worse yet break into the epidural space.

Accidental dural puncture is cause for the immediate termination of saline administration as well as termination of the overall procedure.

14.11. Bleeding at the Entry Point of the Needle and Cannula

The presence of bleeding at the point of introduction of the needle and the cannula is not usually a precursor of complications because this level is above the coccyx. Although bleeding may predispose to infection, such infections are actually rare. The fact that these complications are rare must not lead us to superficiality. In case of some bleeding at the entry point, having first checked that it is not anything serious, one or two stitches may also be required.

14.12. Distension of the Epidural Space

During spinal endoscopy, there is always a certain degree of distension of the epidural space by injection of saline. In the early stages there was little concern about the total volume of normal saline injected in the epidural space during the procedure. Today there is a large consensus among specialists that a volume of 80-100 ml should not be exceeded. It is also recommended that the temperature of the solution be maintained at approximately 37° Celsius to avoid thermal shock. This part of the procedure presents an implied risk, since excess pressure in the epidural space could potentially cause local or distant damage resulting from the pressure creating an obstacle to adequate perfusion (ischemia) of nerve roots or other nerve structures locally or in distant areas (e.g. retina, macula). We must remember also that ischemic consequences are certainly linked to excessive pressure inside the epidural space which in turn was due to the global injected volume of normal saline however also the speed of injection of the saline plays a primary role. The ability to inject at low pressure is always advantageous.

14.13. Presence of Pain during the Procedure

The timely report of pain by the patient explains why it is necessary for the patient to be awake and cooperative throughout the procedure. Pain can be evoked by the passage of the endoscope, the fast injection of saline or might occur after a certain period of time. Usually, in this case, it occurs when the total volume injected is more than 100 ml.

The presence of headache, interscapular pain, neck pain, nausea, vomiting or other discomfort should be considered an indication for terminating the procedure.

14.14. Excessive Insertion of the Endoscope

Another problem relates to the need avoid excessive insertion of the apical end of the spinal endoscope into the spinal canal. During insertion and placement of the endoscope, the discs cannot be recognized or counted to determine the level that is reached. This is especially important since the procedure has an absolute upper limit represented by L2. Currently, only by use of fluoroscopy to guide placement can it be verified that this limit is not exceeded.

This is one of the reasons why we prefer to use flexible endoscopes dedicated to spinal endoscopy rather then using endoscopes that can be used for other purposes. The endoscopes for SE are short therefore, with them, you can not get too high and exceed L2.

In: Manual of Spinal Endoscopy
Editor: Diego Beltrutti

ISBN: 978-1-62257-250-2
© 2012 Nova Science Publishers, Inc.

Chapter 15

Perioperative Management of Thromboprophylaxis and Antithrombotic Therapy

Fabio Intelligente
Chronic Pain Service, Istituti Clinici Humanitas, Rozzano (MI), Italy
Italian School of Pain Medicine (SIMED), Italy

Perioperative management of thromboprophylaxis and antithrombotic therapy is one of the most hot topics in interventional neuroaxial procedures.

Practice guidelines or recommendations available in literature summarize evidence-based reviews and represent the collective experience of recognized experts concerning spinal hematoma related to anticoagulation therapies or thromboprophylaxis in patients who underwent neuroaxial anesthesia or epidural catheter placement but there are no available studies in patients who underwent a spinal endoscopy or endoscopical spinal surgery.

It is generally accepted that elective spine surgeries done through a posterior approach are associated with a very low risk of venous thromboembolism (VTE) In the same manner, we assume spinal endoscopy as a very low risk procedure for thromboembolic events; in fact, spinal endoscopy is performed under local anesthesia, the mean time of the procedure is under 60 minutes and patients are usually fully mobile in a few hours.

Mechanical prophylaxis with compression stockings and an early mobilization of the patient it is considered the first tromboprophylaxis and it should be used in all patients.

If patients do not present any risk factor for a thromoembolism event (VTE), the utility and safety of chemoprophylaxis following a spinal endoscopy is controversial. Low molecular weight heparin (LMWH) or low-dose warfarin, may place patients at an increased risk of symptomatic epidural hematoma and the potential consequences may confound the benefits of these agents.

In patients that present one or more risk factors for VTE (immobility, lower extremity paresis, cancer, previous VTE, postpartum period, drugs intake, genetical, inherited thrombophilias inflammatory bowel disease, nephrotic syndrome, myeloproliferative disorders, hemoglobinuria, obesity, thrombophilia, ecc…) it is mandatory to adopt the mechanical prophylaxis but the utility and safety of chemoprophylaxis should be considered carefully and on an individual case-by-case basis. In each single patient, the agent, dosing regimen, and duration of thromboprophylaxis are based on the identification of risk factors, both individual (eg, age, sex, previous history of thromboembolism) and group-specific (eg, medical illness; immobility, cancer).

On the countrary, in the clinical practice, we often have to treat some patients receiving antithrombotic or antiplatelet therapies for a non-spine related disorder. We know that this kind of medication is potentially related with an elevated risk of spinal hematoma after a spinal procedure. The first step should be to evaluate if it is possible to stop the therapy or if it is necessary to adopt a bridge therapy. It may also be necessary to postpone the procedure in patients where antithrombotic therapy is critical and a suitable "bridge" has not been identified (e.g. drug-eluting stents).

We do not have specific evidence in literature of the incidence of thrombotic events or spinal hematoma in patients who underwent a spinal endoscopy; however, it should be impossible to devise recommendations that will completely eliminate both the risk of spinal hematoma and the risk of thromboembolic events. For such reasons, we adopt some recommendations accredited by the most important American and European societies of anesthesia according to the evidences present in literature about thromboprophylaxis and the risk of spinal hematoma performing neuroaxial block or epidural catheter placement based on case reports, clinical series, pharmacology, hematology, and risk factors for surgical bleeding.

Below, we resume some considerations useful for the perioperative management of the most popular agents used for thromboprophylaxys.

15.1. Antiplatelet Medications

Antiplatelet agents include NSAIDs, thienopyridine derivatives (ticlopidine and clopidogrel), and platelet GP IIb/IIIa receptor antagonists (abciximab, eptifibatide, and tirofiban).

There is no wholly accepted test, including the bleeding time, which will guide antiplatelet therapy.

Usually it is considered prudent to discontinue antiplatelets agents (clopidogrel, acetylsalicylic acid) one week prior to surgery and resume them 24 hours after the procedure.

But observing the pharmacokinetics and the clearance half-life, it should be reasonable to discontinue ticlopidine two weeks prior surgery.

After platelet GP IIb/IIIa inhibitor administration, the time to normal platelet aggregation is 24 to 48 hrs for abciximab and 4 to 8 hrs for eptifibatide and tirofiban, although GP IIb/IIIa antagonists are contraindicated within 4 weeks of surgery.

In patients receiving NSAIDs, there is no contraindication to perform the spinal endoscopy, but it is recommended to discontinue NSAIDs if it is planned to use other medications affecting clotting mechanisms, such as oral anticoagulants, UFH, and LMWH, in the early post-operative period because of the increased risk of bleeding complications.

The discontinuation acetylsalicylic acid is a very controversial issue, most of the anesthesiologist guidelines does not recommend the discontinuation prior to spinal anesthesia or epidural block, but there is no literature about spinal endoscopy.

The controversial concern the aspirin dose-dependent effects: aspirin (and other NSAIDs) may produce opposing effects on the hemostatic mechanism; in fact, platelet cyclooxygenase is inhibited by low-dose aspirin (60-325 mg/d), whereas larger doses (1.572 g/d) will also inhibit the production of prostacyclin (a potent vasodilator and platelet aggregation inhibitor) by vascular endothelial cells and thus result in a paradoxical thrombogenic effect. As a result, low-dose aspirin (81-325 mg/d) is theoretically a greater risk factor for bleeding than higher doses.

15.2. Warfarin

In case of warfarin intake, it should be suspended 5 days before the procedure and the INR value should be inferior to 1.4 at the time of surgery.

Note that in the first 1 to 3 days after discontinuation of warfarin therapy, the coagulation status (reflected primarily by factor II and X levels) may not be adequate for hemostasis despite a decrease in the INR (indicating a return of factor VII activity). Adequate levels of II, VII, IX, and X may not be present until the INR is within reference limits.

Usually, for patients at high risk for thromboembolism, a bridge therapy is required with therapeutic subcutaneous Low molecular wight heparines (LMWH) or intravenous unfractioned heparin (UHF). The LMWH should be discontinued 24 hrs prior surgery and UFH should be discontinued 4 hrs preoperatively.

If it is not indicated to resume warfarin the day after the surgery, therapeutic LMWH will be resumed 24 hrs post-operatively.

15.3. Unfractioned Heparin (UHF)

Anticoagulant effects of UHF is typically monitored with the aPTT, and its effect may be rapidly reversed with protamine administration. The heparin biologic half-life and its anticoagulant effect are both of molecular size and dose-dependent. The major anticoagulant effect of heparin is due to a unique pentasaccharide that binds to antithrombin (AT). Binding of this heparin pentasaccharide to AT accelerates its ability to inactivate thrombin (factor IIa), factor Xa, and factor IXa.

Larger molecular weight heparins will catalyze inhibition of both factor IIa and Xa. Smaller molecular weight heparins will catalyze inhibition of only factor Xa

UFH is administred subcutaneously or intravenously, in both cases, it is suggested to perform neuroaxial procedures at least 4 hrs after the last administration and with aPTT values in the range of normality. After the procedure, resume the heparine at least 1 hour after the procedure but it should be possibly postponed with strict neurological monitoring.

15.4. Low Molecular Weight Heparine (LMWH)

The LMWH biochemical and pharmacologic, clinical properties differ from those of UFH for the lack of monitoring of the anticoagulant response (anti-Xa level), the prolonged half-life, and the lack of irreversibility with protamine.

In the clinical practice, it is commonly administered subcutaneously in the perioperative management of the thromboembolic risk.

In patients receiving low (prophylactic) doses of LMWH, it is recommended to perform the procedure at least 10 to 12 hrs after the last LMWH administration (patients with morning surgeries will need to hold their evening dose the night before). Instead, in patients receiving high (treatment) doses of LMWH (such as enoxaparin 1 mg/kg every 12 hrs oenoxaparin 1.5 mg/kg daily, dalteparin 120 U/kg every 12 hrs, dalteparin 200 U/kg daily), the procedure should be delayed for at least 24 hrs.

After the procedure, usually the prophylactic (low dose) LMWH is restored 8 hrs after the procedure and the second post-operative dose should occur no sooner than 24 hrs after the first dose.

High doses (therapeutic) should be restored at least 24hrs after the procedure. But, if the bleeding risk of the procedure is felt to be high, consideration should be given to administering reduced doses.

15.5. Other Medication such as Rivaroxaban, Thrombin Inibitors (Desirudin, Lepirudin, Bivalirudin, Argatroban)

Until further clinical experience is available, performance of neuraxial techniques is not recommended while taking this medication. Medical literature is still rather poor when we carry out a risk analysis related to the administration of these drugs in relation to neuraxial blocks. Currently we do not recommend performing neuraxial blocks in the process of taking these drugs.

Conclusion

We may consider the spinal endoscopy a minor procedure with low thromboembolism risk and at high risk of major bleeding.

This issue is very complex and at the same time it is one of the most important issues for the right and safe management of the patient. The perioperative management involves balancing the risks of surgical bleeding and thromboembolism because both are potentially catastrophic.

Although the recommendations for management are relatively simple, complexity arises in the determination of who is at "high risk". This evaluation is perhaps best performed within an integrated multidisciplinary clinic by thrombophilia experts.

Each patient is different and a "cookbook" approach is not appropriate. Rather, it can be useful to allow a multidisciplinary evaluation with the hematologist and cardiologist or other specialist experts to optimize the perioperative management for a "tailored" therapy.

Chapter 16

The Risk of Spinal Hematoma

Lorenzo Pasquariello
SSD Pain Medicine, Ospedale Regionale U.Parini, Aosta, Italy
Italian School of Pain Medicine (SIMED), Italy

With the more widespread use of pharmacological prophylaxis of venous thromboembolism, there are also increasing concerns about possible complications that may arise as a result even of minimally invasive procedures into the epidural space in patients taking anticoagulants.

The appearance of a hematoma of the spinal canal in patients undergoing spinal or epidural anesthesia or minimally invasive procedures at the spine is one of the most feared complications. Spinal hematoma, defined as symptomatic bleeding within the spinal neuraxis, is a rare and potentially catastrophic complication of any epidural or spinal procedure because, if not recognized in time, it may result in the appearance of permanent paraplegia. As a result, excessive bleeding into the epidural space may lead to compression, ischemia, nerve trauma, or paralysis.

However, hematoma of the spinal canal is very rare and it is important that the concerns regarding this complication do not lead to denying patients the benefits of an optimal prophylactic, analgesic, or anesthetic procedure in this area.

16.1. The Experience from Epidural Anaesthesia

The true incidence of epidural/spinal hematoma (ESH) is unknown. An analysis performed in Germany in 1993 identified 13 cases of spinal hematoma after 850,000 epidural anesthetics and 7 cases among 650,000 spinal techniques. These data allowed to calculate the incidence of spinal hematoma that was defined less than 1 in 150,000 epidural procedures and less than 1 in 220,000 spinal anesthetics.

During Spinal Endoscopy it is quite frequent that the epidural space becomes a bleeding site; this may occur not only because of the presence of a prominent epidural venous plexus but also as a result of the size of the endoscope and traumatic action exerted by the tool.

Another reason for the apparent increase of spinal hematoma following neuraxial procedures seems to be dependent on the widespread use of LMWH (e.g.: Enoxaparin). This drug has become very popular in many institutions because it provides an effective prophylaxis of DVT. When we refer to what happens in anesthesia we register that the incidence of epidural hematoma formation can increase up to 33:100,000 for epidural anaesthesia and 1:100,000 for spinal anaesthesia.

The medical literature tells us that there are differences between the incidence of ESH in North America and Europe. The most likely explanation for this difference is the variability in dosing between Europe, where the standard dose of LMWH is 4000 units every 24 hours starting 12 hours before the intervention, and the United States, where the dose is 3,000 U every 12 hours starting one hour after surgery. Under certain circumstancies this standard dosing can lead to excessive anti-Xa levels. The risk of spinal bleeding is greater with the use of epidural catheters than with single injection, and a retrospective analysis showed that the incidence of clinically significant spinal bleeding after block using an epidural catheter is in the range of 1:190,000-200,000

Additionally, removing the epidural catheter should be considered a significant risk factor for spinal bleeding, since 30-60% of clinically significant spinal hematomas have occurred after removal of the catheter. Other risk factors are related to technical problems (repeated injections, etc.), anatomical abnormalities, advanced age, the use of anticoagulants and drugs having an anti platelet effect such as NSAIDs. In light of the above data, it should be noted that the guidelines developed by the ESRA (European Society of Regional Anesthesia) show a well-established risk/benefit ratio extrapolated from randomized trials and observational studies. The ASRA (American Society of Regional Anesthesia) has also developed recommendations on "epidural anesthesia and thromboembolic prophylaxis," and these should be consulted for additional details.

In 2003, Vandermeulen reviewed neuraxial procedures with regard to the risk of compressive hematoma within the spinal canal in patients treated with drugs that affect hemostasis (oral anticoagulants or thrombolytic agents). According to the author new preparations such as heparinoids, thienopyridines, glycoprotein IIb/IIIa receptor antagonists, selective inhibitors of factor X, and direct thrombin inhibitors may be used in patients indicated for spinal procedures. However, according to Vandermeulen, it is currently not possible to give specific recommendations for avoiding complications in patients treated with these drugs. The isolated, occasional use of aspirin or NSAIDs does not seem to be a predictor of complications.

The situation is different when these drugs are combined with heparin. In the case of perioperative thromboprophylaxis and of the administration of low molecular weight heparins, it is necessary to allow sufficient time between performing a neuraxial procedure and the previous or subsequent administration of anticoagulant. It is important that heparin drugs are used only at recommended doses. Nevertheless, coagulation tests are required before attempting to perform even a minimally invasive neuroaxial pain procedure in order to confirm that residual effects of the anticoagulants have disappeared. Today the available data about the incidence of ESH after spinal endoscopy are still poor, unclear and ambiguous. They relate to the insertion and removal of epidural catheters. It should be clear that the Spinal Endoscopy procedure is much more traumatic then the insertion of a simple epidural catheter for anesthesia. It follows that the incidence of ESH is certainly equal if not superior to that of epidural anesthesia with epidural catheter. Certainly it cannot be less.

16.2. Risk Factors for the Development of Epidural/Spinal Hematoma

There are several risk factors for the development of an ESH related to the performance of spinal endoscopy. These factors include the following:

- Anatomic abnormalities of the spinal cord or vertebral column
- Vascular abnormalities (such as hypertrophied venous plexus)
- Pathological or medication related alterations in homeostasis
- Alcohol abuse
- Chronic renal insufficiency
- Thick and fibrous adhesions
- Difficult and traumatic insertion of the endoscope
- Size of the endoscope
- Use of laser, biopsy forceps, ...

16.3. Signs and Symptoms of Epidural/Spinal Hematoma

The pain physician must worry and suspect the occurrence of ESH in the presence of the following signs and symptoms that occur in the hours after the end of spinal endoscopy:

- New, acute, sharp LBP
- Sensory and motor loss (numbness and tingling/motor weakness)
- Bowel and bladder dysfunction
- Paraplegia

In: Manual of Spinal Endoscopy
Editor: Diego Beltrutti

ISBN: 978-1-62257-250-2
© 2012 Nova Science Publishers, Inc.

Chapter 17

Historical Considerations

Diego Beltrutti
Chronic Pain Service, Istituti Clinici Humanitas,
Rozzano (MI), Italy
Italian School of Pain Medicine (SIMED), Italy

While the role of endoscopy in the diagnosis and therapy of many pathological conditions has been available for many years and its use has been increasing, the possibility of using an endoscope as a minimally invasive procedure for visualization of the epidural space, spinal cord, and adjacent structures is relatively new. Recent innovations both in fiber optic technology and computer processing of images provides a valuable new tool capable of safely and effectively exploring the anatomical structures contained in the spinal canal. Initial results have been promising and suggest new diagnostic and therapeutic options that are more miniaturized, and thus less intrusive and likely to achieve greater acceptance by patients for treatment of spinal disorders.

However, review of the medical literature shows that attempts at spinal endoscopy have in fact been going on for about 70 years with varying degrees of success. Starting from the pioneering stages, generations of spinal endoscopists have been involved in developing an adequate system that could be easily and safely used in clinical practice. This goal could only recently be achieved with the advent of cold light sources and flexible fiber optic systems for both illumination and image capture.

17.1. Michael Burman

One of the pioneers of this technique was certainly Michael Burman, who was the first to offer direct visualization of the spinal canal and its contents in 1931. Burman removed the spine from 11 cadavers and examined them using a rigid arthroscope with a light source of incandescent bulbs. As can easily be imagined, the diameter of the trocar in which the lamp was mounted was larger than the average width of the spinal canal (about 9.5 mm). Therefore, during visualization, the lenses were not all within the spinal canal. However, in some cases Burman was able to insert the instrument, allowing visualization of anatomical structures contained within the channel such as the dura mater, blood vessels and the *cauda equina*. Because of its width, the endoscope visual field was limited to one inch (2.54 cm). Therefore, Burman concluded that myeloscopy was a procedure limited by available technology.

However, he was convinced that with development of higher quality instruments, in particular, ones that would be characterized by high flexibility and small size, this method could be useful to facilitate post-mortem examinations particularly with reference to the study of *cauda equina*. For this purpose he proposed his Spinascope and the trocar introducer in 1936. Burman did not foresee developments that might suggest mini-invasive therapies in the living subject. He was interested primarily in viewing the contents of the spinal canal in cadavers and the implications of this technique for the diagnosis of spinal infection or tumors.

Since then, endoscopy specialists have proposed new endoscopic instruments every decade or so for use at the level of the spinal canal. A real *in vivo* epidural endoscopy could not be produced until the '80s when the first flexible fiberscope and fiber optics became available. This was a flexible, manageable, secure instrument accepted by clinicians and patients for its reduced size as well as the sharpness of images that could be obtained from the appropriate use of cold light.

17.2. Elias Stern

Elias Stern, of the Department of Anatomy at Columbia University, was among the first to describe a "spinascope," a tool for spinal endoscopy developed as a prototype by American Cystoscope Makers, Inc. The spinascope was designed to examine *in vivo* the content of the spinal canal in a patient undergoing spinal anesthesia in order to gain useful clinical information. Elias Stern probably never used his "spinascope" but foresaw its utility during posterior rhizotomies in patients with intractable pain and anterior rhizotomies in patients with spasticity. He predicted that technological improvements in the construction of these devices would enable endoscopic methodology to replace exploratory laminectomy.

17.3. Lawrence Pool

In 1938, Lawrence Pool published the first clinical use of myeloscopy on anesthetized subjects. The first examination was complicated by the onset of hemorrhage, although he managed to obtain a glimpse of the lumbosacral nerve roots. He subsequently used this technique successfully on seven patients. In one of the first scientific papers on this technique, he reported on these seven patients and his visualization of the *cauda equina* and epidural vessels.

By 1942 Pool had already performed 400 myeloscopies on patients under local anesthesia in the sitting position. These data were published in the journal *Surgery*, and he identified the presence of a number of pathological conditions including primary tumors (neuroepithelioma of the *cauda equina*), metastatic arachnoid adhesions, extruded hernias, and hypertrophy of the *ligamentum flavum* (yellow ligament).

In an era when tools such as CT and MRI were not available, he nevertheless was able to graphically reconstruct what he had seen with myeloscopy. This ability enabled him to confirm or exclude the suggested diagnoses, based on a philosophy of avoiding unnecessary, costly, and risky explorative surgeries.

Despite promising preliminary reports, there wasn't anything else in the medical literature for 30 years. This lack of studies is explained by the failure to develop technological solutions to some of the problems reported by the early clinicians, such as the problem of optical quality of the images given the size of the spinal endoscopes. The industry in those years faced objective technical difficulties in trying to reduce the diameter of the instrument. Other difficulties were also related to the processes of proposal and acceptance in order to have this type of investigation and diagnosis accepted by patients and within the medical profession.

It must be remembered that at Pool's time the technology was not adequate to capture images automatically; lighting was low, precluding use of the equipment available at that time. Consequently, clinicians had to resort to memorization and making drawings by themselves. From Dr. Pool's work, we have his wonderful drawings documenting his observations in the way only a great artist can do.

17.4. Yoshi Ooi

During the '60s and '70s, the Japanese clinician Yoshi Ooi combined the use of hard lenses with a flexible light source. Completely unaware of what the Americans had done, Ooi developed his own endoscope for intra- and extradural examinations, and was the first to use a technology that became available in those years, that of the light source available through fiber optics.

This innovation not only allowed miniaturization of the instrumentation, but also made available a major source of light without being burdened by the risk of the temperature increase associated with incandescent lighting. The fiber optic light source protected the tissues from thermal increase since these fibers absorb infrared rays and reflect visible rays. Miniaturization allowed these myeloscopes to be introduced into the lumbar area and into the interspinous space according to the same percutaneous method used during lumbar epidural anesthesia.

In his first publication, Ooi reported results from 86 patients. The procedure seemed simple and there were no reported serious complications. The availability of a good source of light enabled the permanent recording of these images, and thus the first photographic images in black and white were made available. These images included normal and pathologic anatomy of the lumbar extradural area. The epidural fat tissue, the surface of the dural sac, the *ligamentum flavum*, and the *cauda equina* were photographed in living subjects for the first time.

Ooi did not limit the study to extradural regions, but also performed intradural endoscopies. From 1967 to 1977, he performed a total of 208 procedures, although in some cases there were serious or persistent problems. The main problem related to the procedure was persistent headache caused by dural puncture (reported by 70% of patients).

In the early '80s Ooi and colleagues published an article which described the changes in blood flow in the *cauda equina* during Lasègue's test, the SLR test, and Valsalva's maneuver as seen with the myeloscope. For this study Ooi used a rigid endoscope of 1.8 mm, which was introduced into the intrathecal space. The optical fibers used for this study were used only for the source of light; the endoscopes with optical fibers used both as light source and for image acquisition would not become available until 10 years later.

The author reported changes in blood flow of vessels accompanying the *cauda equina* during the SLR test. During this maneuver, the anterior displacement of the lower *cauda equina* resulted in temporary cessation of blood flow, and he suggested that in some patients this functional condition could be associated with fits of pain.

Additional technological improvements further reduced the diameter of myeloscopes (epiduroscopes). Although these were less invasive, the visual field remained limited. Since better visualization of the epidural space requires an epiduroscope with a diameter of 2.5 mm, epiduroscopy was of limited value in patients affected by spinal stenosis.

At the time of Yoshi Ooi, spinal endoscopy was mainly used for the diagnosis of chronic pain *sine materia*[1], spinal tumors, vascular abnormalities, chronic pain related to inflammation, and fibrosis secondary to surgery. Although during those years clinicians considered the utility of endoscpoy for removal of herniated discs, the technology had not yet been optimized, offering only a rigid endoscope and inadequate light, which increased the difficulty of differentiating healthy tissue from pathologic tissue. In Ooi's time, the possibility of flexible endoscopes was considered, but it took about another 10 years before this dream was realized.

17.5. Rune Blomberg

In the mid-eighties, the Swedish scientist Rune Blomberg described a method for direct visualization of the epidural space. He was interested in studying the anatomical variations of the epidural space with the rationale that this would advance our understanding of the delivery of epidural anesthesia.

Using a small rigid endoscope powered by an optical fiber light source, he showed that the contents of the epidural space differed in relation to the contents of connective tissue and fat tissue. In 12 out of the 30 autopsy studies he conducted, he was able to show how, within the epidural space, visibility was limited by the presence of adhesions. He noted that adhesions between the dura and the *ligamentum flavum* restricted the opening of the epidural space, and that this condition continued despite pressure saline washing. Using an epiduroscope (similar to Stern's spinoscope), Blomberg was also able to see

---

[1] "Sine Mmteria" is a latin phrase meaning that no pathologyhas been found.

from within, the image of a Tuohy needle passing through the *ligamentum flavum* and entering the epidural space. He also showed how an epidural catheter could move within the epidural space according to the local anatomy and based on the presence of obstructions.

With regard to the state of available technology, Blomberg commented that it was *"too early to decide to what extent clinical application is possible with epiduroscopy. Under all circumstances it would be necessary to improve lighting conditions, and to shorten shutter speeds in order to make the method more easily handled."*

In 1989, Blomberg and Olsson performed spinal endoscopy in 10 patients undergoing partial laminectomy for lumbar disc herniation. The authors switched to studies of patients because they believed that some of the conclusions that they reached from examination of cadavers were not generalizable to living subjects. Their concern was the lack of circulation and CSF pressure that was either low or absent; conditions that are very different from those in patients. They demonstrated that the epidural space was a virtual space that opened only after the injection of liquid or air. Blomberg and Olsson confirmed that within the epidural space existed a dorsomedian band of connective tissue that compartmentalized the epidural space. Based on these observations, they suggested that the paramedian approach to the epidural space was safer than the median approach since it provides less risk of bleeding precisely because of the dorsomedian compartmentalization.

We are also indebted to Blomberg for the introduction of another tool useful in the procedure of spinal endoscopy: the videocamera. The combined use of optical fibers for lighting and a computerized system of exposure allowed the author to adequately capture images.

17.6. Koki Shimoji

Shimoji and colleagues in 1991 were the first group to publish their endoscopic experiences using a very small flexible fiber endoscope, with a system of fiber optic lighting instead of a more traditional rigid endoscope. They were able to insert into the epidural and subarachnoid spaces endoscopes with diameters between 0.5 and 1.4 mm. In four cases, they moved the instrument up to the level of the cisterna magna without obvious disturbance to the patients.

Using videocamera technology available at that time, they obtained living visual images including continuous recordings of the endoscopic procedures.

In 10 patients suffering from chronic intractable pain of spinal origin, they inserted the flexible fiber optic myeloscope into the subarachnoid space as well as in the lumbar space through a paramedian approach using a Tuohy needle as the introducer. However, the epidural space was only observed during withdrawal of the instrument, after examination of the subarachnoid space. Visualization of the epidural space was permitted by the passage of a small amount of fluid in the epidural space, allowing a slight relaxation of the space itself. The presence of CSF prevented the tissues of the epidural space from collapsing, and allowed the lens to achieve its focal length of 3-5 mm. However, vision was obstructed in the presence of adherent tissue. Shimoji et al. performed these procedures without sedation of the patients in order to optimally perform sensory evaluations.

Researchers had a strong interest in ascertaining whether the source of chronic pain could be identified by mechanical stimulation. The spinal level where the instrument was positioned was accurately determined through the use of X-rays. In a group of patients with a diagnosis of adhesive arachnoiditis, the nerve roots were observed in the form of a mat, wrapped by filamentous tissue, obscuring visualization of other structural lesions. Nevertheless, three out of five patients who had been diagnosed with adhesive arachnoiditis had a reduction or complete remission of pain following the procedure.

Even if the myeloscope examination could not determine the anatomical cause of pain, the authors concluded that future studies may be able to resolve this issue. Complications were minimal, and were mainly limited to the transient occurrence of post-dural puncture headache and fever, although a few patients also complained of dysesthesia, likely caused by a transient nerve root lesion secondary to an overly rapid removal of the myeloscope.

17.7. Lloyd Saberski and Luke Kitahata

Saberski and Kitahata began in 1991 to evaluate different optical fiber endoscopes in order to determine their suitability for spinal endoscopy. Although there had been significant improvements in technology, the indication of such endoscopes for epiduroscopy had yet to be characterized, since doubts remained regarding whether there were clear advantages relative to non-invasive imaging techniques (CT and MRI). Several technological problems still needed to be resolved in order for spinal endoscopy to achieve a role in clinical practice. One of the problems was related to the focal length of available instruments, since although optical fiber endoscopes had a focal distance of about 2 mm, this was difficult to achieve in a virtual space such as the epidural space. Additionally, there was the need to introduce the endoscope into the epidural space without damage and the requirement for fluoroscopic evaluation of the position of the epiduroscope.

The first optical fiber endoscopes did not have working channels that allowed them to perform biopsies or to administer drugs in a targeted manner. The ideal epiduroscope should be easy to handle, have a working channel, a lens with a very short focal length and/or incorporate a system able to prevent obstruction of the lens by tissues.

Using a caudal approach, Saberski and Kitahata were able to introduce a fiberoptic endoscope in specific areas and to administer steroids in the vicinity of the nerve roots, using an introduction cannula after removing the endoscope. In those years, in order to obtain directionality with the instrument, Kitahata and Saberski introduced the practice of bending the bare optical fiber by gently twisting it around a finger. Then, when it was inserted into the epidural space, they would rotate the proximal end, producing a rotation of the endoscope inside the spinal canal. This maneuver enabled greater visualization of the epidural space.

These early therapeutic successes showed that endoscopy of the spinal canal was not only possible, but also offered the advantage of administering drugs in a targeted manner in the vicinity of specific anatomical structures. This philosophy was very different and even contrary to that of epidural blocks where drug administration follows the path of least resistance.

It was Saberski and Kitahata who suggested the use of saline solution to stretch the epidural space, thereby enabling adequate focal distance for the optical fiber. After injecting an initial volume of 15-20 ml of saline solution, a slight positive pressure was maintained on the syringe in order to achieve optimal distension of the epidural space. The authors also noted that during spinal endoscopy, the nerves that they intended to examine often appeared covered with connective tissue having a "cottony" appearance. The presence of this tissue was not reported by previous researchers, since a more direct approach was generally used, and this approach may have caused bleeding which likely masked this anatomical condition. In contrast, Saberski and Kitahata started the sacral hiatus and reached the target area without interference from bleeding. The "cottony" tissue sometimes seemed to float in saline. With irrigation, it was possible to see that under this cottony tissue there was a dense connective tissue firmly attached to the root, nerves, and adjacent structures. Sometimes it was possible to detect an erythematous aspect of the perineural tissue. These observations were interpreted by the authors as an inflammatory response mediated by the immune system.

17.8. James Heavner

In competition with studies conducted at Yale University, Heavner's group, in 1991, reported their experiences at Texas Tech University using an endoscope inserted into the epidural and subarachnoid space of monkeys, dogs and human cadavers. Their technique was to use a flexible endoscope with an external diameter of 2.1 mm for epidural access and 1.4 mm for intrathecal access. Over the past 20 years Heavner has devoted himself to teaching spinal endoscopy through WIP cadaver courses.

17.9. The Last Twenty Years

In 1992, Möllmann and colleagues published their experiences using a 4 mm rigid endoscope on fresh cadavers. At the Seventh World Congress of the IASP in 1993, Heavner's group used anesthetized dogs to demonstrate the ability to perform spinal endoscopy from the sacral hiatus to the cervical level without major technical difficulties or cardiovascular responses. However, they nevertheless concluded that there was still a need for further technological improvements before the clinical potential of spinal endoscopy could be realized. Also using anesthetized dogs, Rosenberg in 1994 demonstrated the potential of a new flexible endoscope with a deflective tip.

In 1994, Schutze and Kurtz published their experiences performing spinal endoscopy in 12 patients suffering from various painful conditions. They were able to show normal and pathologic anatomic structures, including important areas of fibrosis and adhesions in two patients with Failed Back Surgery Syndrome (FBSS). Using endoscopic control, they were able to implant three epidural catheters in a targeted manner.

17.10. Current Clinical Perspectives

To summarize the historical perspective, it is possible to characterize three crucial and distinct stages in the development of spinal endoscopy:

1) The ability to produce cold light at a sufficiently bright intensity
2) The miniaturization of endoscopes to more sizes appropriate for spinal endoscopy
3) The introduction of more flexible materials

As mentioned above, it was not until the '90s that a system for using a fiber optic endoscope with a flexible cord was available. Although the three points mentioned all contributed to enhancing this technique, it was mainly the flexibility of the instruments and the decision to use the caudal route that enabled consistent clinical use in humans.

Although these instruments were veritable jewels of technology, they had some limitations that had to be resolved before obtaining more widespread acceptance and use.

An improvement in the control system was needed, as well as the presence of one or more working channels by which instruments such as biopsy forceps, lasers, and radiofrequency sources could be passed through for specific procedures.

In response to these needs, several companies including Catheter Imaging Systems, Inc. (CIC), Myelotec Inc., Clarus, Karl Storz, and Equip Medikey have developed and/or produced different instruments that have been used for spinal endoscopy since the 90s.

Since 1996, spinal endoscopy has been increasingly used to administer steroids targeted to nerve roots. The original technique of Saberski and Kitahata has gradually evolved based on the work of many international clinicians, eventually enabling procedures including lysis of epidural adhesions by volumetric injection, lasers or radiofrequency generators, and by the mechanical action of a Fogarty-type balloon.

In the medical population there is a deep-rooted belief that the targeted administration of local anesthetics and/or steroids by spinal endoscopy is superior to percutaneous techniques of epidural block with local anesthetics and steroids. However, randomized controlled trials (RCTs) have not been performed.

Starting in 1998, several variants of the original technique became available. Therefore some American insurance companies began to evaluate whether the medical literature would support reimbursement of these procedures. Many concluded that there was insufficient scientific support in the medical literature (no studies such as RCTs) and therefore they classified spinal endoscopy an experimental procedure. This classification made the procedure ineligible for reimbursement to the doctors and centers where it was performed.

Although there was considerable interest to continue research in spinal endoscopy, a number of factors prevented its progress.

Some believe that Myelotec, in those years the leading company in the marketing of epiduroscopes, was the victim of a vicious cycle. In other words, the crisis of spinal endoscopy in those years seems closely related to issues raised in this leading company. By someone it has been suggested that, they thought that through initial sales they could increase the resources available to expand research as well as the number and quality of studies.

But at this time, American health policy decision-makers ("managed care") slowed down the expansion of spinal endoscopy and reduced the funds available for clinical trials and research. However, it is also true that it was very difficult to initiate RCT studies, even if research funds had been available. Many patients were not interested in participating in clinical studies of "experimental" techniques, and they opted for surgery or endoscopy based on individual preferences and clinical circumstances.

The demands by insurance companies to base therapy and payment decisions on the availability of results from RCTs seemed particularly strict for endoscopy, considering that other minimally invasive techniques and surgical procedures were performed in the U.S. with a scarcity of outcomes data. Since the technique of spinal endoscopy is easy to perform and relatively safe, it made sense to suggest its use before considering a surgical spinal procedure, especially for conditions of chronic pain such as FBSS. In order to do so, however, it would have been necessary to re-educate doctors, patients, surgeons and insurance companies to this new paradigm.

Spinal endoscopy with flexible fiberscopes has opened up new pathophysiologic and therapeutic horizons. Before Saberski, McCarron and Saals, pain conditions related to the presence of a disc disease were solely attributed to nerve compression. Since there was no knowledge that disc disease and spinal pain could be due to the presence of an inflammatory condition controlled by the immune system, this interpretation was not even considered. The prevailing attitude in the medical profession was still based on a mechanical interpretation that was generally related to the size of the disc herniation as observed by MRI. The pain was interpreted as being related to the size of the herniation and its mechanical effect. This particular theory that the magnitude of the hernia determined the pain intensity continued for many years and was still in vogue during the '90s.

Today we know that the chemical regulation of cellular signals, in combination with changes in CNS receptivity, determine the experience of pain. Pain is real and organic, and a patient may be totally debilitated due to pain and suffering even if the hernia is small.

The '90s ended with several studies that reported on the benefits of spinal endoscopy. These included anatomical studies in living subjects; the risk of dural puncture during combined anesthesia techniques; and changes of epidural anatomy after epidural anesthesia.

In Germany, Shutze published his experiences from 139 patients using spinal endoscopy to position epidural catheters.

In the '90s there were also numerous publications describing clinical cases that highlighted the potential of endoscopic programs. Spinal endoscopy has been used in cases of both acute and chronic pain in different ways and for different diseases. This is easily understood since a multitude of different pathophysiologic conditions result in spinal pain.

Recently, Saberski suggested that spinal pain can be independent of compression factors, and may be representative of a "leaky disc syndrome" or of an autoimmune response. It is thus possible that in the near future, back pain will be able to be treated with specifically targeted chemotherapeutic interventions at the epidural level.

While there have been discussions, there is still a lack of evidence about which environmental factors, infections, could influence the immune system response to antigens/chemicals. Animal studies are being conducted in an attempt to analyze the cellular signals and immune responses, and their results, when available, will define many common afflictions of the spine such as medical and non-surgical diseases.

In 1999, Richardson published a review of endoscopy in the British Journal of Anaesthesia. In a study published in 2000, Saberski retrospectively evaluated the outcomes of patients treated by either laminectomy or epidural endoscopy for pain due to simple disc compression. He reported that 72% of subjects treated using spinal endoscopy went back to work, while only 28% of those treated with laminectomy returned to work. Moreover, consumption of opiates was significantly lower in the group of patients treated by spinal endoscopy.

In the same year, at a conference at the World Foundation for Pain held in New York, Saberski reported that the medical costs for treatment of acute disc herniation using spinal endoscopy were lower than the costs of treatment by laminectomy/discectomy. Additionally, the subjects treated by spinal endoscopy returned were more likely to return to work than those treated using laminectomy/discectomy.

In 2001, Richardson et al. published their experiences treating a group of 34 patients, 17 of whom suffered from post-laminectomy syndrome (FBSS). In all cases, the fibrous material in the epidural space was reduced after one year from surgery. In the same time frame it was shown an improvement in indicators of stability as well as of pain measures by VAS. In 2001 two publications by Manchikanti et al. demonstrated excellent short-term response using endoscopic techniques for adhesiolysis. Even after 12 months, the positive effects were maintained in 22% of the subjects. Comparable results were also reported by Krasuski et al.

In 2005 Raffaeli and Righetti published their experience with the use of Resablator (a surgical device using a particular kind of radiofrequency that can be used through the working channel of the epiduroscope) in an attempt to ameliorate spinal pain due to FBSS.

In 2005 Manchicanti and Coll. studied 50 patients in a prospective, randomized, double-blind trial to determine the outcome of spinal endoscopic adhesiolysis to reduce pain and improve function and psychological status in patients with chronic refractory low back and lower extremity pain. A total of 83 patients were evaluated, with 33 patients in Group I and 50 patients in Group II. Group I served as the control, with endoscopy into the sacral level without adhesiolysis, followed by injection of local anesthetic and steroid. Group II received spinal endoscopic adhesiolysis, followed by injection of local anesthetic and steroid. Among the 50 patients in the treatment group receiving spinal endoscopic adhesiolysis, significant improvement without adverse effects was shown in 80% at 3 months, 56% at 6 months, and 48% at 12 months. The control group showed improvement in 33% of the patients at one month and none thereafter.

Based on the definition that less than 6 months of relief is considered short-term and longer than 6 months of relief is considered long-term, a significant number of patients obtained long-term relief with improvement in pain, functional status, and psychological status. The authors concluded that spinal endoscopic adhesiolysis with targeted delivery of local anesthetic and steroid is an effective treatment in a significant number of patients with chronic low back and lower extremity pain without major adverse effects.

We can summarize and conclude this chapter by stating that current techniques of spinal endoscopy using flexible optical fiber endoscopes were strongly stimulated by advances in technology. This journey has taken more than 70 years and much progress has been made since the early efforts by

Burman. Although we certainly hope for further advances that will make epiduroscopes more manageable, more versatile, and with a higher optical resolution, spinal endoscopy has shown that it has an important role in the diagnostic and therapeutic armamentarium of Pain Clinicians.

In: Manual of Spinal Endoscopy
Editor: Diego Beltrutti

ISBN: 978-1-62257-250-2
© 2012 Nova Science Publishers, Inc.

Chapter 18

Consensus Conference on Spinal Endoscopy

Diego Beltrutti
Chronic Pain Service, Istituti Clinici Humanitas,
Rozzano (MI), Italy
Italian School of Pain Medicine (SIMED), Italy

On September 17, 1998 in Iserlohn, and on October 3rd, 1998 in Bad Durkheim, an international group of experts formulated a document entitled "Standards for Epiduroscopy." The scientific basis for these recommendations for the use of epiduroscopy included studies published in the specialized medical literature and on the clinical experience of the participants: O. Groll (Dortmund, Germany), J.E. Heavner (Lubbock, Texas, USA), H. Kurtz (Bad Durkheim, Germany), H.J. Leu (Zurich, Switzerland), M. Möllmann (Munster, Germany), N.A. Rawal (Orebro, Sweden), L. Saberski (New Haven, Connecticut, USA), and G. Schutze (Iserlohn, Germany).

The participants in this international working group agreed on the following general principles for administering the clinical application of endoscopy of the spinal canal.

Endoscopy of the spinal canal, also known as Epiduroscopy, was defined as a minimally invasive percutaneous endoscopic investigation of the epidural space that allows color visualization of the anatomical structures inside the spinal canal: dura mater, blood vessels, connective tissue, nerves, fat and pathologic structures such as adhesions, fibroses, inflammation, and stenotic changes.

The general guidelines established for the use of endoscopy of the spinal canal were:

- Diagnosis and treatment of spinal pain syndromes
- Observation of pathology and anatomy
- Direct and targeted application of drugs
- Direct lysis of scar tissue through the use of drugs, atraumatic dissection, laser and other instruments
- Positioning of epidural catheters and of electrocatheters for spinal cord stimulation (SCS) via epidural or subarachnoid insertion (subarachnoid intrathecal catheters connected to a subcutaneous "port" or to totally implanted pumps for infusion of opioids or baclofen)
- In addition to minimally invasive surgery

18.1. Italian Interest Group on Epiduroscopy

As far as Italy is concerned, on March 16, 2004 a group of medical experts in pain medicine and epiduroscopy met in Treviso to discuss the need to establish precise guidelines for the procedure itself and to start a National Interest Group on Epiduroscopy under the aegis of the World Society of Pain Clinicians (WSPC) and the International Neuromodulation Society (NSI). In attendance were: Alberto Alexandre (Treviso), William Raffaeli (Rimini), Marzia Rocco (Castelfranco Emilia), Claudio Reverberi (Cremona), Lorenzo Pasquariello (Aosta), Diego Beltrutti (Alba-Bra), Fabrizio Micheli (Piacenza), Vincenzo Firetto (Ancona), Giuliano De Carolis (Pisa), and Attilio Di Donato (Roma).

At the meeting, the international consensus document mentioned above ("Standards for Epiduroscopy") was discussed and unanimously approved by all meeting participants.

Several important needs were also identified, including choosing a site as the official organ of the Italian Working Group on Epiduroscopy (www.epiduroscopia.com) in order to gain wider recognition of the technique and of the Pain Centers associated with the interest group. The meeting participants also expressed the need to provide clear, qualified and realistic answers to the pressing questions of many patients regarding this technique, as well as the need to define a document of informed consent that could be adopted at all centers for submission to patients who are candidates for spinal endoscopy.

The meeting also considered the urgency for creating opportunities for training in Italy to properly educate those who were willing to learn the procedure, since there is currently no specialty in Pain Medicine at the University level and these minimally interventional pain procedures are not considered in the specialization schools for neurosurgery, orthopedics or anesthesiology.

However, it was also considered that training in SE should be limited to colleagues in various specialized areas (anesthesia/pain management, neurosurgery, orthopedics) who have an appropriate academic and professional curriculum, including the mastery of other techniques of interventional pain therapy and primary work experience in the field of pain.

18.2. The GILE Group

In December 2004, several members of the National Interest Group on Epiduroscopy established "GILE" (Gruppo Italiano di Lavoro sull' Epiduroscopia, or in English, Italian Working Group on Epiduroscopy) which has as the sole objective providing specialist physicians with a solid theoretical base in spinal endoscopy using e-learning.

Entrusted to this project were Dr Diego Beltrutti (Alba-Bra), Dr. Attilio Di Donato (Roma), Dr. Lorenzo Pasquariello (Aosta), and Dr. Valentino Menardo (Cuneo). A special program was activated with courses connected with the Italian School of Pain Medicine (www. Simed.net).

18.3. The WISE Group

On 3rd and 4th March 2006, a group of internationally recognized experts in spinal endoscopy met in Graz (Austria). This group was composed of Andreas Sandner-Kiesling (A), Günther Weber (A), Günter Schütze (D), Diego Beltrutti (I), Gerbrand J. Groen (NL), and Lloyd Saberski (USA). They established the World Initiative on Spinal Endoscopy (WISE), and in the two-days of the meeting, the group produced a document defining the various aspects of spinal endoscopy, including the following purposes:

1. As a diagnostic tool

   - in the case of diagnosis of clinically relevant epidural pathologies. This can occur when the pain can be attributed to the structures of the epidural space (spinal canal) on the basis of medical history, physical examination, laboratory tests and current imaging
   - when biopsy of epidural structures is needed for histopathology and histochemical tests
   - in order to perform stimulation and provocative tests (e.g. electrical, mechanical, light) of the nervous structures

2. As a support tool

   - in the case of precise placement of epidural or spinal catheters
   - for precise positioning of spinal cord stimulation (SCS) electrodes
   - as visual and technical support during minimally invasive surgery
   - for removal of foreign bodies

3. As a therapeutic tool

   - to irrigate the epidural space (epidural wash out with normal saline)
   - for direct application of therapeutic agents (Racz's mixture, steroids, anesthetics, …)
   - to determine lysis of adhesions/scar tissue (mechanical, pharmacological, laser, RF) under direct visualization

The document not only considers technical and clinical problems of spinal endoscopy, but also the need for quality control on the entire procedure. It is strongly recommended that patients receive comprehensive information on the technique prior to providing consent.

A structured and detailed protocol should be developed to insure adequate data collection during spinal endoscopy procedures, and the procedure itself should be videotaped for both educational and medico-legal purposes. It is also suggested that a specific position be created, that of creation of a central control procedure (data manager) to verify that the various centers adhere to the recommendations of WISE regarding indications and patient selection.

The acquisition of data must include at least: the type of epiduroscope used, the type and amount of fluids administered, the duration of the procedure, side effects and complications.

WISE also requires that documented and accredited training must precede any attempt to perform spinal endoscopy, although these parameters have yet to be fully defined.

We reiterate the need for relevant industry support in producing materials for spinal endoscopy and to provide financial sponsorship aimed at education and training of clinicians while maintaining scientific independence. WISE is available to organize cadaver courses for those who already have a basic knowledge of the technique.

In: Manual of Spinal Endoscopy
Editor: Diego Beltrutti

ISBN: 978-1-62257-250-2
© 2012 Nova Science Publishers, Inc.

Chapter 19

Essential Equipment

Diego Beltrutti
Chronic Pain Service, Istituti Clinici Humanitas,
Rozzano (MI), Italy
Italian School of Pain Medicine (SIMED), Italy

Spinal endoscopy is a complex procedure. In addition to manual adjustments by the clinician and knowledge of intrathecal imaging, it requires the availability of specific equipment including:

19.1. Digitized Fluoroscope (DF)

Il provides a mobile system for the production of digital images in real time (Figure 1) resulting from the interaction of X-rays with the patient. DF relies on the same basic principles as conventional fluoroscopy, but is improved by the addition of computer technology.

The DF contains an image intensifier that transforms the radiologic image into a luminous image; an optical coupling system and a video camera that produce an electronic video signal from the image emitted from of the intensifier tube; an analogue-to-digital converter that transforms the analogue signal into appropriate frequencies using Fourier transformation.

The DF is part of a mobile console consisting of the display and image processing components, a computer, and memory.

In this unit, the presence of different microprocessors ensures the operation of the various subsystems and data storage.

The system allows for crisp, undistorted images that can be stopped or enlarged without losing resolution, speeding up the examination itself, and allows storage in an optical or magneto-optical format.

19.2. Surgical Table with Radiotransparent Platform

It does not interfere with fluoroscopic imaging since it consists of a platform of carbon fiber to allow passage of x-rays (Figure 2). Common surgical beds are not sufficient as they have a frame and metal brackets which limit fluoroscopic imaging.

The possibility of lateral supports allows the operator to intervene with the patient in lateral decubitus. Moreover, the bed must be shaped to allow easy rotation of the C arch of the fluoroscope.

19.3. Endoscopic Video Column

This term refers to the mobile cart on which is placed the set of equipment used during the procedure, such as the monitor, cold light source, power supply for the video camera, and the video recorder and connecting systems (Figure 3).

The optical part of the endoscope is in turn connected to the camera.

19.4. Flexible Spinal Endoscope

As shown in Figures 4, 5 and 6, it consists of the ocular, sterile protection tube of the optic fibers, and the handle to direct the flexible tip of the endoscope in the desired direction.

The endoscope can be equipped with a non- sterile optic fiber when using the EPI-C endoscope, and must be equipped with a sterile optic fiber with use of any other spinal endoscopes.

Essential Equipment

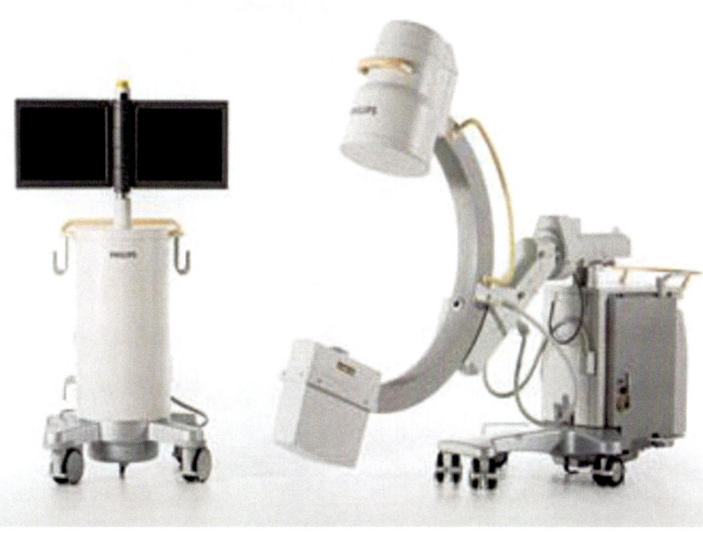

Figure 1. Example of high quality portable fluoroscopy. You can see the two moving parts: the C-arm and the memory unit with dual monitor and printer.

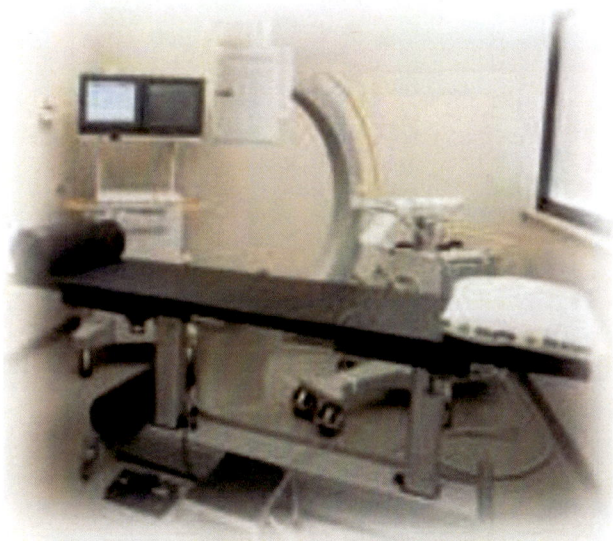

Figure 2. Example of a surgical table with radio transparent platform. The absence of side rails, metal frame and brackets is crucial, especially when it is necessary to use oblique views.

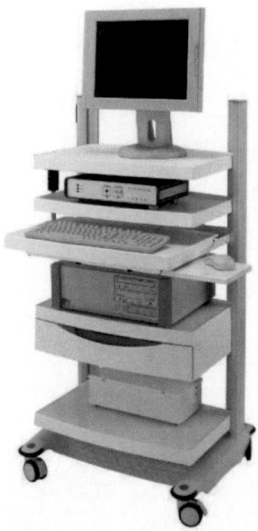

Figure 3. The endoscopic video column.

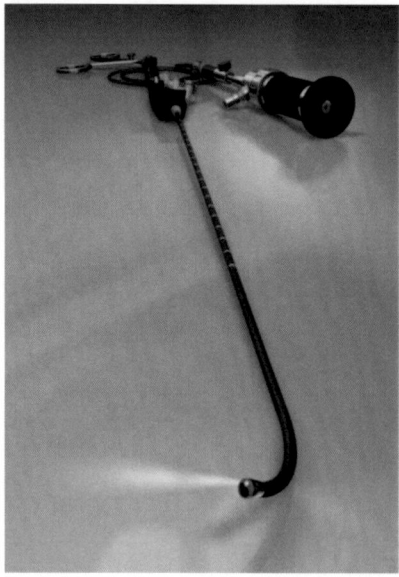

Figure 4. EPI-C Equip Medikey flexible spinal endoscope. You can see here the various components: the ocular, optics, the protection tube for the optic fiber (in blue), handle, the video guide with access to the two working channels (one for tools and the other for irrigation).

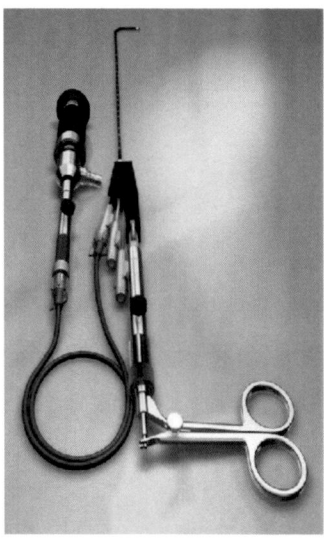

Figure 5.This picture shows the handle that makes possible the movement and flexion of the tip.

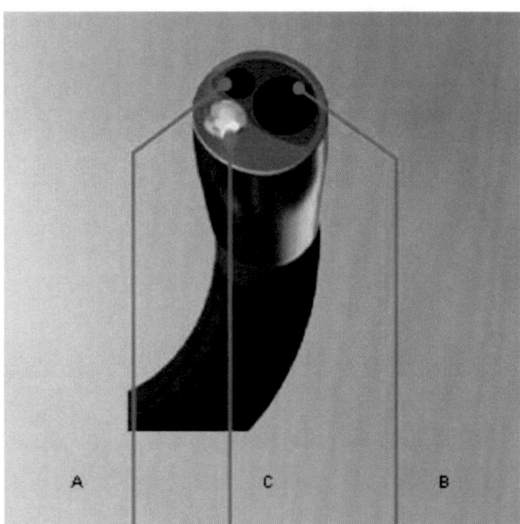

Figure 6. Details of the tip of the EPI-C Equip Medikey video guide. In this image you can clearly see the lens (C) which distally seals the channel of the optic fiber. This lens prevent the release of the optic fiber outside the video guide. Therefore it can not penetrate into the spinal canal. For this reason it is not necessary to sterilize the optic fiber. A and B respectively indicate the irrigation channel (0,6 mm) and the working channel (1,2 mm).

Chapter 20

Materials

Attilio Di Donato
Anaesthesia and Pain Medicine Service,
Ospedale Concordia per Chirurgie Speciali, Roma, Italy
Italian School of Pain Medicine (SIMED), Italy

The following equipment is required when performing an ESS procedure:

- Equipment for radiation protection (leaded coat, thyroid collar protector, goggles). The authors are used to wear Epimed leaded gloves. It is also advisable to wear a radiation detector under the glove of the most exposed hand.
- Woven non woven (WNW) sterile gown, hat and mask
- Sterile gloves, worn on top of the leaded gloves. Some clinicians have told us that leaded gloves are an encumbrance, and therefore many clinicians claim that they do not use them because they reduce manual sensitivity.
- Sterile towels: we recommend a WNW set specifically meant for epiduroscopy procedure

1 - EPI-C Equip Medikey video guide (Figures 20.1) for spinal endoscopy

1 - 17 GA Tuohy needle. We use and suggest epidural needles such as the flexible Introducer Cannula (SCA) over a 17 GA Tuohy needle. For more expert clinicians we suggest the RX coudé epidural needle[1]

1 - Disposable scalpel with fine tip (blade 10)

1 - 5 ml syringe with short needle for 2% lidocaine (local anesthetic); it will be used to create a button of anesthesia (bolus) at the sacral hiatus.

1 - 10 ml syringe for administration of the contrast agent Metrizamide (Amipaque) 300; the contrast agent is not mandatory but can be used if the clinician deems it necessary.

1 - 2.5 ml syringe for injection of steroid (Triamcinolone 40 mg).

1 - 10 ml syringe for saline administration (a volume exceeding 60 ml must not be left in the epidural space).

1 - saline drip of 100 ml for the antibiotic to be infused 30 minutes before the procedure.

1 - 10 ml syringe with Naropin (Ropivicaine) 0.2%; a small quantity of the anesthetic can be injected into the epidural space to make the procedure more tolerable; from 4 to 6 ml. Some clinicians prefer to use Lidocaine because the injection of local anesthetic also allows to value the presence of a dural tear. In this case a spinal anesthesia will appear in minutes.

1 - suture package (gauze, needle holders, scissors, surgical forceps, small Klemmer forceps)

- Silk "00" for suturing the skin

20.1. Advantages

Hygienic: the presence of a "disposable" catheter with a single terminal lens in combination with a reusable optic fiber eliminates problems of contamination.

Excellent vision: the EPI-C® spinal fiberscope has a single terminal lens that does not come out from the catheter and does not require sterilization. This construction enables good imaging over a long period of time by eliminating the damage to the fiber optic components that may occur during the sterilization process.

---

[1] These needles are produced by Epimed Int. USA.

Ease of flexion: built-in mechanisms allow compensation when the endoscope encounters the need for specific angular flexation.

Small external diameter: 2.65 mm (8F)

Very large working channel: 1.2 mm (3.6F) that enables use of a variety of instruments including biopsy forceps, RF, and laser fiber systems.

Separate irrigation channel: 0.6 mm (1.9F)

Ease of use: since the lighting cable and the camera head are in a separate holder, there is no longer a need to provide support structures for these components.

Repairs: factory repairs have become obsolete, since repairs or changes to the optical system or its parts, if necessary, can be done directly by the medical staff.

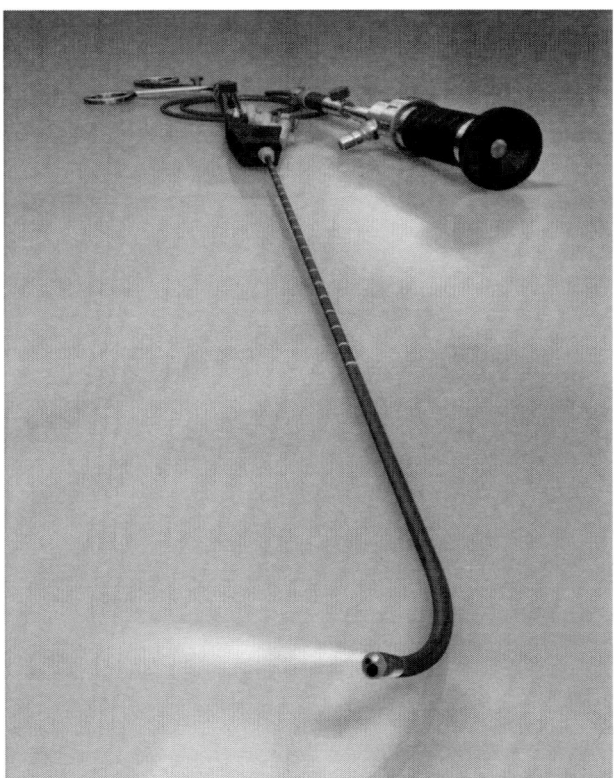

Figure 20.1. The EPI-C® fiberscope from Polydiagnost for spinal endoscopy is the first disposable instrument which combines the imaging quality of a re-usable with the safety of a disposable one.

20.2. Cost Considerations

No upkeep: Since the EPI-C® spinal endoscope is "disposable," factory repairs, repair costs, and down-time without an endoscope are eliminated. Any necessary repairs can be performed by the medical staff directly in the operating room, providing both convenience and cost-savings.

Superior reliability: the EPI-C® optical system is very reliable, which saves time and costs. Tests carried out on these lenses have shown that no maintenance was needed even after more than 100 uses.

Cost containment: the EPI-C® flexible endoscope has an innovative design that allows the entire system to be available at a much lower price than the similar systems on the market. If we consider the global costs ("disposable" catheters) and compare them with the competitive systems, the EPI-C® system saves more than 30%.

20.3. Technical Data

Ø2.65 mm endoscopic catheter (8 F) with a tip flexible up to 90°.
Working Channel 1: Ø 1.2 mm (3.6 F)
Working channel 2: Ø 0.6 mm (1.9 F)

Catheter lengths: 30 cm and 42 cm. All catheters have markings that indicate their length in order to easily monitor their position.

Even with inserted instruments, the EPI-C® epiduroscope can be bent up to 180°. The torsion resistance of the catheter enables the rotation to reach every location. The tip is softly rounded for gentle access into narrow spaces

20.4. Optical System

The optical system varies from 6000 to 10000 pixels depending on the model, allowing optimal transmission of images and an equally optimal transport of light in order to maintain perfect lighting of the area to be examined.

The EPI-C® Spinal Endoscope is the first "disposable" endoscope that combines the image quality of a reusable endoscope with the security of a "disposable." Because of its main feature, integration of the lens and catheter, it is not necessary to sterilize the optical fiber and therefore it will have a long working life. This instrument of spinal endoscopy has a special and revolutionary design which allows the operator to work with a safe and always "transparent" tool. The affordable cost of the instrument enables purchase by any Pain Center.

In: Manual of Spinal Endoscopy
Editor: Diego Beltrutti

ISBN: 978-1-62257-250-2
© 2012 Nova Science Publishers, Inc.

Chapter 21

Future Trends

Diego Beltrutti
Chronic Pain Service, Istituti Clinici Humanitas,
Rozzano (MI), Italy
Italian School of Pain Medicine (SIMED), Italy

Because of advances in spinal endoscopic procedures enabling its wider clinical application, we will need to find answers to certain questions that are currently emerging in the light of experience gained over the years.

21.1. Is Spinal Endoscopy Really an Irreplaceable Diagnostic and Therapeutic Tool?

The first question refers to the added value of spinal endoscopy compared with other common imaging techniques. In other words, can we be sure that this procedure can really provide more detailed anatomical and clinical information relative to non-invasive imaging techniques in general use such as CT or MRI? Will its use for targeted epidural administration of steroids and local anesthetics under endoscopic guidance result in better outcomes than the traditional epidural administration of steroids? Are the results of adhesiolysis obtained with a catheter placed under spinal endoscopy really better than the positioning of the catheter implanted with the sole use of fluoroscopy?

From preliminary data it would seem that these questions can be answered in an affirmative way. However these questions are still awaiting an unequivocal answer, since it is difficult to provide clinical evidence in the absence of appropriate RCTs. For a variety of reasons, these studies have not yet been performed, but it is hoped that they will be done in the near future to help resolve the above issues.

In recent years, spinal endoscopy technology has made great progress. Technological research in industry and academics have provided clinicians with endoscopes having a substantially smaller diameter, greater flexibility, and working channels to introduce laser, RF instruments and biopsy forceps. This reduction in external diameter is especially important since it results in a less invasive technique.

If the miniaturization of instruments and use of optic fibers on one hand is a definite advantage, on the other hand this reduction can be considered to decrease the visual field the image quality. With the reduction in the diameter of the optic fiber it is clear that the visual area is limited and this does not help us during positioning, and a technological solution in needed for this problem.

In the past, image quality was often very poor and was a deterrent to the widespread use of this technique. In recent years, digital and computer technology have been of great help. We expect that in the near future there will be additional improvements in image quality through the introduction of image processors capable of reconstructing magnified and crisp images that were originally small and not always clear.

Another improvement occurred in the acquisition and image processing. In recent years there has been a sharp increase in the number of pixels available, and most likely this tendency will continue in the future. The availability of new videocameras, digital image processing, and use of computers are all factors that have contributed to spinal endoscopy advancing from being mainly a diagnostic procedure to becoming an important micro-invasive analgesic technique.

It would also be crucial, especially for educational purposes, to initiate a database with typical univocal images, representing different normal and pathologic states. The availability of an atlas of endoscopic images both normal and pathological would help increase precision and reduce ambiguity for when writing reports or describing results.

We are confident that in the near future, spinal endoscopy will be considered a valuable technique and will be increasingly used for the resolution of cases of chronic radiculopathy in where there is a discrepancy among the finding of the various evaluations (patient report, imaging, neurophysiological tests). With increasing use and recognition, spinal endoscopy is gaining a role of great importance in the diagnostic and therapeutic instruments of clinical pain.

21.2. Thecaloscopy

After years of studies and research on the endoscopy of the epidural space, a new technique has been recently proposed for the visualization of the sub arachnoid space and the thecal sac. This new technique of endoscopy is thecaloscopy.

Thecaloscopy is a percutaneous procedure involving the use of a flexible endoscope introduced into the sub arachnoid space. It allows the direct visualization of the lumbar subarachnoidal space for diagnostic and therapeutic purposes.

Warnke JP and collegues in 2003 treated twelve patients with this new technique. Arachnoid cysts were successfully fenestrated and an intraspinal meningocoele treated with endoscopic assistance. Authors concluded that thecaloscopy is a safe procedure, when skilfully performed, that provides an opening for a wide range of new diagnostic and therapeutic options.

Thecaloscopy should be able to solve cases of arachnoiditis, a clinical painful condition chracterized by the inflammation of the meninges and subarachnoid spaces. The presence of a lumbar arachnoiditis may lead to complete obliteration of the nerve root sleeves, to the adherence of nerve roots between them, to the aggregation of nerve roots in the proximity of the *cauda equina*. In arachnoiditis the cause of adhesions may be idiopathic or secondary to infectious diseases, tumors, surgical procedures in the spine (such as spinal surgery).

In: Manual of Spinal Endoscopy
Editor: Diego Beltrutti

ISBN: 978-1-62257-250-2
© 2012 Nova Science Publishers, Inc.

Chapter 22

Conclusion

Diego Beltrutti
Chronic Pain Service, Istituti Clinici Humanitas,
Rozzano (MI), Italy
Italian School of Pain Medicine (SIMED), Italy

The desire to develop an endoscopic procedure for direct visualization of the spinal canal is over seventy years old. However, only in the last ten years have technological developments allowed the practical realization of this dream. The knowledge and the instruments available today represent the work of many researchers, although the technique has only recently been appropriately developed, improved, and refined so that this technique can be widely and safely used.

Nevertheless, RCT studies are still needed to fully characterize the advantages of this technique relative to other imaging techniques (e.g. MRI and CT) and procedures that are routinely used to administer drugs in the epidural space. In other words, the exact role of spinal endoscopy in the diagnostic and therapeutic procedures of painful conditions of the spine has not yet been clearly defined.

Three dimensional examination of the epidural space and anatomical structures contained therein, in real time and in direct view, allows identification of epidural diseases and can be of great help in locating the generators of persistent spinal pain. However we feel able to say that this ability to identify and study diseases of the epidural space using a minimally invasive procedure, together with the possibility of targeted drug administration is not offered by any other technique available today.

Only in the future we will know whether spinal endoscopy will maintain the promise shown as an effective and minimally invasive therapy for radicular pain and other forms of disabling and debilitating spinal pain.

Other therapeutic options offered by this new methodology include the removal of intra-and extra-dural scar tissue, drainage of cysts, precise positioning of SCS electrodes, targeted and video guided biopsies, studies of cellular biology and of inflammatory mediators and retrieval of foreign bodies (e.g. removal of pieces of epidural catheters, spinal catheters, and broken epidural electrodes).

Today, many researchers are convinced that the possibility of blocking inflammatory mediators in order to modify inflammatory processes that underly multiple and protean tissue reactions holds great promise as a therapeutic approach.

In conclusion, we can say that the spinal endoscopy, beyond its value as diagnostic technique, can be used safely and effectively in the therapy and removing of epidural scar tissue, to administer drugs in specific areas and under direct visualization. Also there is the possibility to perform biopsies, also under direct visualization, allowing through this procedure to more precisely define the underlying disease.

This also applies to the video guided installation of catheters (e.g. Versa-Kath®, Poli-Kath® epidural catheters), electro catheters for spinal cord stimulation (SCS) in specific areas of the epidural space.

Spinal endoscopy is a fascinating procedure that opens new windows on the diagnosis and treatment of those pathologic conditions accessible through the epidural space.

References

[1] Amirikia A; Scott IU; Murray TG; Halperin LS. Acute bilateral visual loss associated with retinal hemorrhages following epiduroscopy. *Arch Ophthalmol,* 2000 118, 287-289.

[2] Anderson SR; Racz GB; Heavner J. Evolution of epidural lysis of adhesions. *Pain Physician,* 2000 3, 262-270.

[3] Avellanal M; Diaz-Reganon G. Interlaminar approach for epiduroscopy in patients with failed back surgery syndrome. *Br J Anaesth,* 101, 244-249.

[4] Beltrutti D; Raffaeli W. Preliminary report on radio frequency myeloscopy (RFM) with "R-Resablator" in the management of failed back surgery syndrome pain. In: Hanaoka K, Yuge O, Namiki A, Editors. *11th International Pain Clinic World Society of Pain Clinicians.* Bologna: Medimond; 2004; 333-337.

[5] Beltrutti D. Towards a consensus document on percutaneous epiduroscopy. In: Beltrutti D, Varrassi G, Editors. *12th International Pain Clinic World Society of Pain Clinicians.* Bologna: Medimond; 2006; 223-226.

[6] Bergqvist D; Lindblad B; Matzsch T. Risk of combining low molecular weight heparin for thromboprophylaxis and epidural or spinal anesthesia. *Semin Thromb Hemost, 1993* 19 Suppl 1,147-151.

[7] Blomberg R. A method for epiduroscopy and spinaloscopy. Presentation of preliminary results. *Acta Anaesthesiol Scand,* 1985 29, 113-116.

[8] Blomberg R. The dorsomedian connective tissue band in the lumbar epidural space of humans: an anatomical study using epiduroscopy in autopsy cases. *Anesth Analg,* 1986 65, 747-752.

[9] Blomberg RG; Olsson SS. The lumbar epidural space in patients examined with epiduroscopy. *Anesth Analg,* 1989 68,157-160.
[10] Blomberg RG. Epiduroscopy and spinaloscopy: endoscopic studies of lumbar spinal spaces. *Acta Neurochir,* 1994 61 Suppl, 106-107.
[11] Blomberg RG.: Technical advantages of the paramedian approach for lumbar epidural puncture and catheter introduction. A study using epiduroscopy in autopsy subjects. *Anaesthesia,* 1988 43, 837-483.
[12] Bogduk N. Management of chronic low back pain. *Med J Aust,* 2004 180, 79-83.
[13] Bosscher HA; Heavner JE. Incidence and severity of epidural fibrosis after back surgery: an endoscopic study. *Pain Practice,* 2010 1,18-24.
[14] Boswell MV; Trescot AM; Datta S; et Al. Interventional techniques: evidence-based practice guidelines in the management of chronic spinal pain. *Pain Physician,* 2007 10, 7-111.
[15] Broadman LM. Non-steroidal anti-inflammatory drugs, antiplatelet medications and spinal axis anesthesia. *Best Pract Res Clin Anaesthesiol,* 12005 9, 47-58.
[16] Burman MS. Myeloscopy or the direct visualization of the spinal canal and its contents. *J Bone Joint Surg,* 1931 13, 695-696.
[17] Chao CC; Hu S; Ehrlich L; Peterson PK. Interleukin-1 and tumor necrosis factor-alpha synergistically mediate neurotoxicity: involvement of nitric oxide and of N-methyl-D-aspartate receptors. *Brain Behav Immun* 1995 9: 355-365.
[18] Chatani K; Kawakami M; Weinstein JN; et Al. Characterization of thermal hyperalgesia, c-fos expression, and alterations in neuropeptides after mechanical irritation of the dorsal root ganglion. *Spine,* 1995 20, 277-289.
[19] Dashfield AK; Taylor MB; Cleaver JS; Farrow D. Comparison of caudal steroid epidural with targeted steroid placement during spinal endoscopy for chronic sciatica: a prospective, randomized, double-blind trial. *Br J Anaesth,* 2005 94, 514-519.
[20] Devulder J; Bogaert L; Castille F; et Al. Relevance of epidurography and epidural adhesiolysis in chronic failed back surgery patients. *Clin J Pain,* 1995 11, 147-150.
[21] Di Ieva A; Barolat G; Tschabitscher M; et Al. Lumbar arachnoiditis and thecaloscopy: brief review and proposed treatment algorithm. *Cen Eur Neurosurg,* 2010 71, 207-212.

[22] Di Donato A; Pasquariello L; Beltrutti D. *Manuale di endoscopia spinale: Una via nuova per la diagnosi e la terapia dei dolori cronici del rachide.* Cuneo: Isimed; 2008.

[23] Donato AD; Fontana C; Pinto R; Beltrutti D; Pinto G.The effectiveness of endoscopic epidurolysis in treatment of degenerative chronic low back pain: a prospective analysis and follow-up at 48 months. *Acta Neurochir,* 2011 108 Suppl, 67-73.

[24] Epter RS; Helm S II, Hayek SM, et Al. Systematic review of percutaneous adhesiolysis and management of chronic back pain in post lumbar surgery syndrome. *Pain Physician,* 2009 12, 361-378.

[25] Fai KR; Engleback M; Norman JB; Griffiths R. Interlaminar approach for epiduroscopy in patients with failed back surgery syndrome. *Br J Anaesth,* 2009 102, 280-281.

[26] Fibuch EE. Percutaneous epidural neuroplasty: cutting edge or potentially harmful pain management? Reg Anesth Pain Med, 1999 24,198-201.

[27] Fonoff ET; de Oliveira YS; Lopez WO; et Al. Endoscopic-guided percutaneous radiofrequency cordotomy. *Neurosurg.* 2010 113, 524-527.

[28] Fonoff ET; Lopez WO; de Oliveira YS; et Al. Endoscopic approaches to the spinal cord. *Acta Neurochir,* 2011 108 Suppl, 75-84.

[29] Franz S; Dadak AM; Moens Y; et Al. Use of endoscopy for examination of the sacral epidural space in standing cattle. *Am J Vet Res,* 2008 69, 894-899.

[30] Geurts JW; Kallewaard JW; Richardson J; Groen GJ. Targeted methylprednisolone acetate/hyaluronidase/clonidine injection after diagnostic epiduroscopy for chronic sciatica: a prospective, 1-year follow-up study. *Reg Anesth Pain Med,* 2002 27, 343-352.

[31] Gill JB; Heavner JE. Visual impairment following epidural fluid injections and epiduroscopy: a review. *Pain Med,* 2005 6, 367-374.

[32] Gillespie G; MacKenzie P. Epiduroscopy-a review. *Scott Med J,* 2004 49, 79-81.

[33] Hanai F; Matsui N; Hongo N. Changes in responses of wide dynamic range neurons in the spinal dorsal horn after dorsal root or dorsal root ganglion compression. *Spine,* 1996 21, 1408-1414.

[34] Hayek SM; Helm S; Benyamin RM; et Al. Effectiveness of Spinal Endoscopic Adhesiolysis in post lumbar surgery syndrome: a systematic review. *Pain Physician,* 2009 12, 419-435.

[35] Heavner JE; Bosscher H; Dunn D; Lehman T. Xanthosis in the spinal epidural space-an epiduroscopy finding. *Pain Pract,* 2004 4, 39-41.

[36] Heavner JE; Bosscher HA; Wachtel MS. Cell types obtained from the epidural space of patients with low back pain/radiculopathy. *Pain Pract*, 2009 9, 167–172.

[37] Heavner JE; Racz GB; Raj P. Percutaneous epidural neuroplasty: prospective evaluation of 0.9% NaCl versus 10% NaCl with or without hyaluronidase. *Reg Anesth Pain Med*, 1999 24, 202-207.

[38] Heavner JE; Wyatt DE; Bosscher HA. Lumbosacral epiduroscopy complicated by intravascular injection. *Anesthesiology*, 2007 107, 347-350.

[39] Hirsh J; Bauer KA; Donati MB; et Al. Parenteral anticoagulants: American College of Chest Physicians Evidence-Based Clinical Pract Guidelines (8th Edition). *Chest*, 2008 133, 141S-159S.

[40] Holmstrom B; Rawal N; Axelsson K; Nydahl PA. Risk of catheter migration during combined spinal epidural block: percutaneous epiduroscopy study. *Anesth Analg*, 1995 80, 747-753.

[41] Horlocker TT; Heit JA. Low molecular weight heparin: biochemistry, pharmacology, perioperative prophylaxis regimens, and guidelines for regional anesthetic management. *Anesth Analg*, 1997 85, 874–885.

[42] Horlocker TT; Wedel DJ; Benzon H; et Al. Regional anesthesia in the anticoagulated patient: defining the risks (the second ASRA Consensus Conference on Neuraxial Anesthesia and Anticoagulation). *Reg Anesth Pain Med*, 2003 28,172-197.

[43] Horlocker TT; Wedel DJ; Rowlingson JC. Regional anesthesia in the patient receiving antithrombotic or thrombolytic therapy American Society of Regional Anesthesia and Pain Medicine evidence-based guidelines (Third Edition). *Reg Anesth Pain Med*, 2010 35, 64-101.

[44] Igarashi T; Hirabayashi Y; Shimizu R; et Al. Thoracic and lumbar extradural structure examined by extraduroscope. *Br J Anaesth*, 1998 81, 121-125.

[45] Igarashi T; Hirabayashi Y; Shimizu R; et Al. The epidural structure changes during deep breathing. *Can J Anaesth*, 1999 46, 850-855.

[46] Igarashi T; Hirabayashi Y; Shimizu R; et Al. The fiberscopic findings of the epidural space in pregnant women. *Anesthesiology*, 2000 92,1631-1636.

[47] Igarashi T; Hirabayashi Y; Seo N; et Al. Lysis of adhesions and epidural injection of steroid/local anaesthetic during epiduroscopy potentially alleviate low back and leg pain in elderly patients with lumbar spinal stenosis. *Br J Anaesth*, 2004 93, 181-187.

[48] Jalali S. Epidural endoscopic adhesiolysis: A valuable technique in treating refractory low back and extremity pain. *Am J Anesthesiol*, 2000 27, 261-264.
[49] Van Boxem K; Cheng J; Patijn J; et Al. Lumbosacral radicular pain. *Pain Pract*, 2010 10, 339-358.
[50] Kessel G; Bocher-Schwarz HG; Ringel K; Perneczky A. The role of endoscopy in the treatment of acute traumatic anterior epidural hematoma of the cervical spine: case report. *Neurosurgery*, 1997 41, 688-690.
[51] Kitahata LM. Recent advances in epiduroscopy. *J Anesth*, 2002 16, 222-228.
[52] Kitamura A; Sakamoto A; Aoki S; et Al. Epiduroscopic changes in patients undergoing single and repeated epidural injections. *Anesth Analg*, 1996 82, 88-90.
[53] Koes BW; Scholten RJ; Mens JM; Bouter LM. Efficacy of epidural steroid injections for low-back pain and sciatica: a systematic review of randomized clinical trials. *Pain*, 1995 63, 279-288.
[54] Komiya K; Igarashi T; Suzuki H; et Al. In vitro study of patient's and physician's radiation exposure in the performance of epiduroscopy. *Reg Anesth Pain Med*, 2008 33, 98-101.
[55] Krasuski P; Poniecka AW; Gal E; et Al. Epiduroscopy: Review of technique and results. *Pain Clinic*, 2001 13, 71-76.
[56] Lahad A; Malter AD; Berg AO; Deyo RA. The effectiveness of four interventions for the prevention of low back pain. *Jama*, 1994 272, 1286-1291.
[57] Manchikanti L; Bakhit CE. Percutaneous lysis of epidural adhesions. *Pain Physician*, 2000 3, 46-64.
[58] Manchikanti L; Boswell MV; Rivera JJ; et Al. A randomized, controlled trial of spinal endoscopic adhesiolysis in chronic refractory low back and lower extremity pain. *BMC Anesthesiology*, 2005 5,10.
[59] Manchikanti L; Pakanati RR; Bakhit CE; Pampati V: Role of adhesiolysis and hypertonic saline neurolysis in management of low back pain: evaluation of modification of the Racz protocol. *Pain Digest*, 1999 9, 91-96.
[60] Manchikanti L; Pampati V; Bakhit CE; Pakanati RR. Non-endoscopic and endoscopic adhesiolysis in post-lumbar laminectomy syndrome: a one-year outcome study and cost effectiveness analysis. *Pain Physician*, 1999 2, 52-58.

[61] Manchikanti L; Pampati V; Fellows B; et Al. Effectiveness of percutaneous adhesiolysis with hypertonic saline neurolysis in refractory spinal stenosis. *Pain Physician,* 2001 4, 366-373.

[62] Manchikanti L; Pampati V; Fellows B; et Al. Role of one day epidural adhesiolysis in management of chronic low back pain: a randomized clinical trial. *Pain Physician* 2001 4, 153-166.

[63] Manchikanti L; Saini B; Singh V. Spinal endoscopy and lysis of epidural adhesions in the management of chronic low back pain. *Pain Physician,* 2001 4, 240-265.

[64] Manchikanti L; Singh V. Epidural lysis of adhesions and myeloscopy. *Curr Pain Headache Rep,* 2002 6, 427-435.

[65] Manchikanti L; Singh V; Cash KA ; et Al. A comparative effectiveness evaluation of percutaneous adhesiolysis and epidural steroid injections in managing lumbar post surgery syndrome: a randomized equivalence controlled trial. *Pain Physician,* 2009 12, E355-368.

[66] Manchikanti L; Singh V; Cash KA; et Al. Management of pain of post lumbar surgery syndrome: one-year results of a randomized, double-blind, active controlled trial of fluoroscopic caudal epidural injections. *Pain Physician,* 2010 13, 509-521.

[67] McCarron RF, Wimpee MW, Hudkins PG, Laros GS: The inflammatory effect of nucleus pulposus. A possible element in the pathogenesis of low-back pain. *Spine (Phila Pa 1976),* 1987 12, 760-764.

[68] Merrill DG; Rathmell JP; Rosenquist RW. Epiduroscopy and epidural steroid injections. [letter] *Anesthesiology,* 2008 108, 538; author reply 108, 538.

[69] Mizuno J; Gauss T; Suzuki M; et Al. Encephalopathy and rhabdomyolysis induced by iotrolan during epiduroscopy. *Can J Anaesth,* 2007 54, 49-53.

[70] Mollmann M; Holst D; Enk D; et Al. [Spinal endoscopy in the detection of problems caused by continuous spinal anesthesia]. *Anaesthesist,* 1992 41, 544-547.

[71] Morisot P: [Is posterior lumbar epidural space partitioned?] Ann Fr Anesth Reanim, 1992 11, 72-81.

[72] Mourgela S; Anagnostopoulou S; Sakellaropoulos A; et Al. Endoscopic anatomy of the thecal sac using a flexible steerable endoscope. *J Neurosurg Sci,* 2007 51, 93-98.

[73] Nash TP. Epiduroscopy for lumbar spinal stenosis. [letter] *Br J Anaesth,* 2005 94, 250; author reply 250-1.

[74] NASS. *Evidence-based clinical guidelines for multidisciplinary spine care*. Burr Ridge (IL): North American Spine Society (NASS); 2009; 96.
[75] Olmarker K; Rydevik B. Pathophysiology of sciatica. *Orthop Clin North Am,* 1991 22, 223-233.
[76] Ooi Y; Mita F; Satoh Y. Myeloscopic study on lumbar spinal canal stenosis with special reference to intermittent claudication. *Spine (Phila Pa 1976),* 1990 15, 544-549.
[77] Ooi Y; Satoh Y; Inoue K; et Al. Myeloscopy, with special reference to blood flow changes in the cauda equina during Lasegue's test. *Int Orthop,* 1981 4, 307-311.
[78] Pool JL. Direct visualization of dorsal nerve roots of the cauda equina by means of a myeloscope. *Arch Neurol,* 1938 39,1308-1312.
[79] Pool JL. Myeloscopy: intraspinal endoscopy. *Surgery,* 1942 11,169-182.
[80] Racz GB; Heavner J; Raj P. Epidural neuroplasty. *Semin Anesth Periop Med Pain,* 1997 16, 302-312.
[81] Racz GB; Noe C; Heavner JE. Selective spinal injections for lower back pain. *Curr Rev Pain,* 1999 3, 333-341.
[82] Raffaeli W; Righetti D. Surgical radio-frequency epiduroscopy technique (R-ResAblator) and FBSS treatment: preliminary evaluations. *Acta Neurochir,* 2005 92 Suppl:121-125.
[83] Raffaeli W; Righetti D; Andruccioli J; Sarti D. Periduroscopy: general review of clinical features and development of operative models. *Acta Neurochir,* 2011 108 Suppl, 55-65.
[84] Raj PP. Evolution of interventional techniques. *Agri* 2004 16, 25-34.
[85] Richardson J; McGurgan P; Cheema S; et Al. Spinal endoscopy in chronic low back pain with radiculopathy. A prospective case series. *Anaesthesia,* 2001 56, 454-460.
[86] Richardson J. Realizing visions. *Br J Anaesth,* 1999 83, 369-371.
[87] Rodgers A, Walker N, Schug S, et Al.: Reduction of postoperative mortality and morbidity with epidural or spinal anaesthesia: results from overview of randomised trials. *Brit Med J,* 2000 321, 1493.
[88] Ross JS, Robertson JT, Frederickson RC, et Al.: Association between epidural scar and recurrent radicular pain after lumbar discectomy: magnetic resonance evaluation. *Neurosurgery,* 1996 38, 855-861.
[89] Rowlingson JC; Hanson PB. Neuraxial anesthesia and low-molecular-weight heparin prophylaxis in major orthopedic surgery in the wake of the latest American Society of Regional Anesthesia Guidelines. *Anaesth Analg,* 2005 100, 1482-1488.

[90] Ruetten S; Meyer O; Godolias G. Application of holmium:YAG laser in epiduroscopy: extended practicabilities in the treatment of chronic back pain syndrome. *J Clin Laser Med Surg*, 2002 20, 203-206.

[91] Ruetten S; Meyer O; Godolias G. Endoscopic surgery of the lumbar epidural space (epiduroscopy): results of therapeutic intervention in 93 patients. *Minim Invasive Neurosurg*, 2003 46,1-4.

[92] Saal JA. Spinal injections: past, present and future. *Spine J*, 2001 1, 387-389.

[93] Saberski LR; Brull SJ. Spinal and epidural endoscopy: a historical review. *Yale J Biol Med*, 1995 68, 7-15.

[94] Saberski LR, Gerena F: Safety of epidural endoscopy. Reg Anesth Pain Med, 1998 23, 324-325.

[95] Saberski LR; Kitahata LM. Direct visualization of the lumbosacral epidural space through the sacral hiatus. *Anesth Analg*, 1995 80, 839-840.

[96] Saberski LR; Kitahata LM. Review of the clinical basis and protocol for epidural endoscopy. *Conn Med*, 1996 60, 71-73.

[97] Saberski LR. A retrospective analysis of spinal canal endoscopy and laminectomy outcomes data. *Pain Physician*, 2000 3, 193-196.

[98] Saberski LR. Comment on epiduroscopic changes in patients undergoing single and repeated epidural injections. *Anesth Analg*, 1996 83, 661.

[99] Saitoh K; Igarashi T; Hirabayashi Y; et Al. [Epiduroscopy in patients with chronic low back pain without remarkable findings on magnetic resonance imaging] *Masui*, 2001 50,1257-1259.

[100] Schofferman J; Reynolds J; Herzog R; et Al. Failed back surgery: etiology and diagnostic evaluation. *Spine J*, 2003 3, 400-403.

[101] Schütze G; Kurtze H. Direct observation of the epidural space with a flexible catheter-secured epiduroscopic unit. *Reg Anesth Pain Med*, 1994 19, 85-89.

[102] Schütze G. *Epiduroscopy: spinal endoscopy.* Heidelberg: Springer Verlag; 2008.

[103] Shah RV; Heavner JE. Recognition of the subarachnoid and subdural compartments during epiduroscopy: two cases. *Pain Pract*, 2003 3, 321-325.

[104] Shimoji K; Fujioka H; Onodera M; et Al. Observation of spinal canal and cisternae with the newly developed small-diameter, flexible fiberscopes. *Anesthesiology*, 1991 75, 341-344.

[105] Schroeder DR. Statistics: detecting a rare adverse drug reaction using spontaneous reports. *Reg Anesth Pain Med*, 1998 23,183–189.

[106] Slipman CW; Shin CH; Patel RK; et Al. Etiologies of failed back surgery syndrome. *Pain Med,* 2002 3, 200-214.
[107] Smuck M; Benny B; Han A; Levin J. Epidural fibrosis following Percutaneous Disc Decompression with coblation technology. *Pain Physician,* 2007 10, 691-696.
[108] Stern EL. The Spinascope; a new instrument for visualizing the spinal canal and its contents. *Medical Record (NY),* 1936 143, 31-32.
[109] Sugawara O; Atsuta Y; Iwahara T; et Al. The effects of mechanical compression and hypoxia on nerve root and dorsal root ganglia. An analysis of ectopic firing using an in vitro model. *Spine,* 1996 21, 2089-2094.
[110] Tobita T; Okamoto M; Tomita M; et Al. Diagnosis of spinal disease with ultrafine flexible fiberscopes in patients with chronic pain. *Spine (Phila Pa 1976),* 2003 28, 2006-2012.
[111] Tryba M. Epidural regional anesthesia and low molecular heparin: pro. *Anasthesiol Intensivmed Notfallmed Schmerzther,* 1993 28, 179–181.
[112] Tryba M; Wedel DJ. Central neuraxial block and low molecular weight heparin (enoxaparine): lessons learned from different dosage regimes in two continents. *Acta Anaesthesiol Scand,* 1997 111 Suppl, 100-104.
[113] Tryba M: European practice guidelines: thromboembolism prophylaxis and regional anesthesia. *Reg Anesth Pain Med,* 1998 23,178-182.
[114] Uchiyama S; Hasegawa K; Homma T; et Al. Ultrafine flexible spinal endoscope (myeloscope) and discovery of an unreported subarachnoid lesion. Spine (Phila Pa 1976), 1998 23, 2358-2362.
[115] van Tulder MW; Koes BW; Bouter LM. Conservative treatment of acute and chronic nonspecific low back pain. A systematic review of randomized controlled trials of the most common interventions. *Spine (Phila Pa 1976),* 1997 22, 2128-2156.
[116] Vandermeulen E. Guidelines on anticoagulants and the use of locoregional anesthesia. *Minerva Anestesiol,* 2003 69, 407-411.
[117] Waldman SD. Epiduraloscopy. In: Waldman SD, editor. *Atlas of Interventional Pain Management.* 2nd Ed. Philadelphia: Saunders; 2004; 568-572.
[118] Warnke J. P; Köppert H; Bensch-Schreiter B; et Al. Thecaloscopy part III: First clinical application. Minimally Invasive Neurosurg 2003 46, 94-99.
[119] Warnke JP, Di X, Mourgela S, Nourusi A, Tschabitscher M: Percutaneous approach for thecaloscopy of the lumbar subarachnoidal space *Minim Invasive Neurosurg* 2007 50,129-131.

[120] Warnke JP; Tschabitscher M; Nobles A. Thecaloscopy: the endoscopy of the lumbar subarachnoid space, part I: historical review and own cadaver studies. *Minim Invasive Neurosurg* 2001 44, 61-64.
[121] Wulf H; Striepling E. Postmortem findings after epidural anaesthesia *Anaesthesia,* 1990 45, 357-361.
[122] Wulf H. Epidural anaesthesia and spinal haematoma. *Can J Anaesth,* 1996 43,1260-1271.

Acknowledgments

Whenever a writing project is completed, authors are duly bound to thank someone. In this case the word "grateful" is indispensable, because the idea of writing this book goes back a few years and the actual process was postponed several times for different reasons. Understandably, with its completion we have the joy of having created this Manual on Spinal Endoscopy which we hope will be helpful for young colleagues who decide to take this technique.

This would not have been possible without the encouragement of the Italian School of Pain Medicine (SIMED), a private organization who is careful and nurturing in the advancement of Pain Medicine. Without their support, we would never have been be able to propose a text on a niche subject such as spinal endoscopy, a procedure currently used by fewer than a hundred Italian pain experts.

Thanks are also addressed to our friends and colleagues in pain medicine Valentino Menardo MD and Enrico Obertino MD of the Pain Centre of ASO Santa Croce and Carle (Cuneo), who helped to create the iconography of this volume.

I cannot forget Jay Bienen, psychologist and friend who gave me his willingness and his precious time to read the text in order to improve our English.

Thanks also go to our families who supported us and understood the reasons for our frequent absences and shortcomings during the writing and production of this volume.

And last but not least, a special thank you to our patients from whom we have learned a lot and for whom we are still studying.

Diego Beltrutti

Contributors

Dr. Diego Beltrutti
Chronic Pain Service,
Istituti Clinici Humanitas,
Rozzano (Mi), Italy

Dr. Attilio Di Donato
Anaesthesia and Pain Medicine Service,
Ospedale Concordia per Chirurgie Speciali,
Roma, Italy

Dr. Fabio Intelligente
Chronic Pain Service,
Istituti Clinici Humanitas,
Rozzano (Mi), Italy

Dr. Lorenzio Pasquariello
SSD Pain Medicine,
Ospedale Regionale U. Parini,
Aosta, Italy

Index

A

accidental dural puncture, 74
adhesiolysis, 127
advantages, 114
analgesia, 27
antibiotic, 71
antibiotic prophylaxis, 71
antiplatelet agents, 79
antiplatelet medications, 79
antithrombotic therapy, 77
arachnoid cysts, 121
arachnoiditis, 21
argatroban, 81
arthroscopy, 3, 9

B

bivalirudin, 81
bleeding at the entry point, 75
Blomberg, Rune, 91
bronchoscopy, 9
Burman, Michael, 88

C

cerebral vascular diseases, 63
chronic persistent headache, 64
Clarus Spine Scope, 6
coccyx, 15
colonoscopy, 9
colposcopy, 10
complex cases, 36
consensus conference, 101
conservative treatment, 133
contraindications, 63, 64
cost considerations, 116
cost containment, 116
Creutzfeldt-Jakob disease, 58, 59, 60
cystoscopy, 10

D

decompression, xii, 133
desirudin, 81
digitized fluoroscope, 107
direct nerve injury, 74
direct visualization, 131, 132
disesthesia, 72
disposable scalpel, 114

E

ease of flexion, 115
ease of use, 115

EGD, 10
endoscopic biopsy, 10
endoscopic images, 45
endoscopic video column, 108
EPI-C Spinal Endoscope, 7
epidural fat, 49
epidural fibrosis, 133
epiduroscopy, 1, 4, 101, 102, 103, 126, 127, 129, 130, 132
epilepsy, 63
ERCP, 10
excellent vision, 114
excessive insertion, 76

F

factory repairs, 115
Flexible spinal endoscope, 108
fluoroscopy, 45

G

general anesthesia, 63, 65
GILE group, 102

H

heparin, xii
Heavner, James, 95

I

imaging, xii, 23, 96
inability to maintain a prone position, 63
inadequate equipment, 64, 66
inadequate training, 64, 66
indications, v, 31, 33
infections, 73
Italian interest group on epiduroscopy, 102

K

Karl Storz Epiduroscope (KSE), 6
Karl Storz Epiduroscope FLEX - X^2, 7
Karl Storz Miniature Epiduroscope, 6
Kitahata, Luke, 93

L

lack of consensus, 64
laparoscopy, 3, 11
laringoscopy, 11
laser fiber systems., 115
laser, xii, 132
lepirudin, 81
local anesthesia, 27
low molecular weight heparin, 81

M

malformations, 64
mechanical prophylaxis, 78
metrizamide (amipaque), 114
monitoring, 27
Myelotec NaviCath, 6
Myelotec Video Guided Catheter, 6

N

needle malpositioning, 68
no upkeep, 116

O

Ooi, Yoshi, 90
open tip spinal endoscopes, 61
optical system, 116

P

pain during epidural injection, 72

pain medicine, ix, x, 1, 5, 9, 13, 17, 19, 25, 31, 37, 45, 53, 57, 63, 67, 77, 83, 87, 101, 103, 107, 113, 119, 123, 128, 135
paresis and paralysis, 74
patient positioning, 29
patient preparation, 28
patient selection, 32
periduroscopy, 1, 131
perioperative management, 77
persistent headache, 71
persistent unexplained radiculopathy, 34
pharmacotherapy, 26
Pool, Lawrence, 89
practice guidelines, 77
pregnancy, 64, 65
presence of septic lesions, 64
previous brain surgery, 64
prions, 58
proctoscopy, 3, 11
proctosigmoidoscopy, 11
puncture and aspiration, 35

R

radiotransparent platform, 108
RCT studies, 97, 123
renal insufficiency, 65
retinal diseases, 64
retinal hemorrhages, 72
RF, 3, 34, 51, 120
rivaroxaban, 81

S

Saberski, Lloyd, 93
sacral hiatus, 15
saline, 72
sedation, 27
Shimoji, Koki, 92
sigmoidoscopy, 11
somato sensorial evoked potentials, 25
somatoform disorders, 64
spinal cord stimulation, xii, 2
spinal cord, 65

spinal endoscope, 5
spinal endoscopy, 1, 3, 15, 21, 28, 33, 34, 35, 47, 63, 66, 97, 98, 107, 124, 130, 131
spinal hematoma, 83
sterility, 28
sterilization, 59, 60
Stern, Elias, 88
superior reliability, 116
surgical table, 108

T

targeted positioning of epidural catheters, 34
Tarlov cysts, 34
technical data, 116
technique, 37
thecaloscopy, 121
thoracoscopy, 11
thrombin inhibitors, 81
thromboprophylaxis, 77
triamcinolone, 114
Tuohy needle, 6, 92, 93

U

unfractioned heparin (UHF), 80
unrealistic expectations, 64
unstable angina, 64

V

visual support, 35

W

warfarin, 80
Wireless capsule endoscopy, 11
WISE group, 102
Wolf Epiduroscope, 7
woven non woven (WNW), 113